FEAR OF HUMILIATION

FEAR OF HUMILIATION

Integrated Treatment of Social Phobia and Comorbid Conditions

Edited by
W. Walter Menninger, M.D.

JASON ARONSON INC.
Northvale, New Jersey
London

The original source of this material is the *Bulletin of the Menninger Clinic,* Spring 1994, vol. 58, no. 2, suppl. A. Copyright © 1994 The Menninger Foundation.

The editorial staff of the *Bulletin of the Menninger Clinic* wishes to express appreciation to the following for granting permission to excerpt from or adapt portions of previously published material: American Psychological Association, Guilford Press, and Dr. David H. Barlow.

10 9 8 7 6 5 4 3 2 1

Library of Congress Cataloging-in-Publication Data

Fear of humiliation : integrated treatment of social phobia and
  comorbid conditions / W. Walter Menninger, editor.
      p. cm.
    "Supplement to the Bulletin of the Menninger Clinic, vol. 58, no.
2, suppl. A, spring, 1994."
    Material presented on May 22, 1994 at the Annual Meeting of the
American Psychiatric Association in Philadelphia, Penn.
    Includes bibliographical references and index.
    ISBN 1-56821-465-0
    1. Social phobia—Congresses. 2. Social phobia—Complications—
Congresses. I. Menninger, W. Walter. II. American Psychiatric
Association. Meeting (147th : 1994 : Philadelphia, Pa.)
III. Bulletin of the Menninger Clinic, Vol. 58, No. 2 (Supplement A)
    [DNLM: 1. Depressive Disorder—therapy—congresses. 2. Phobic
Disorders—therapy—congresses. 3. Comorbidity—congresses.
4. Fear—congresses. WM 178 F2885 1995]
RC552.S62F43 1995
616.85'225—dc20
DNLM/DLC
for Library of Congress   94-49180

Manufactured in the United States of America. Jason Aronson Inc. offers books and cassettes. For information and catalog write to Jason Aronson Inc., 230 Livingston Street, Northvale, New Jersey 07647.

Contents

Acknowledgments

The material contained in *Fear of Humiliation: Integrated Treatment of Social Phobia and Comorbid Conditions* was presented on May 22, 1994, at the annual meeting of the American Psychiatric Association in Philadelphia, Pennsylvania, at an educational symposium sponsored by Menninger. The symposium was chaired by W. Walter Menninger, MD. Both the symposium and these published proceedings were supported by an unrestricted educational grant from Roche Laboratories, a member of the Roche Group.

Introduction

Philip R. Beard, MDiv, MA

Social phobia is an underrecognized—and thus undertreated—psychiatric disorder. Although identified as a clinical entity nearly three decades ago, it was not included in the *Diagnostic and Statistical Manual of Mental Disorders* until 1980. Moreover, reports on in-depth studies of social phobia did not appear in the literature until 1985.

Given the manifold and potentially severe consequences of social phobia, one may wonder why this condition has escaped intense psychiatric scrutiny until the past decade. As the chapters in this volume attest, social phobia is often intermingled in complex ways with a host of other psychiatric disorders, including related phobias, anxiety disorders, eating disorders, depression, personality disorders, and alcohol and drug abuse and dependence. The other, apparently more disabling, disorder often receives primary attention. The challenge, therefore, is to disentangle the various factors that contribute to interpersonal anxiety—sometimes crystallized as social phobia, often intertwined with comorbid conditions.

Fear of Humiliation seeks to sharpen diagnostic perception of this often-disabling disorder. The authors also describe in some detail the current array of treatment modalities—psychodynamic, cognitive-behavioral, and pharmacological—with emphasis on the need for integrated treatment.

Kathryn Zerbe offers a psychodynamic perspective on social phobia. Acknowledging that the psychodynamic literature has neglected this condition, she presents two case examples to illustrate how shame, aggression, trauma, and unresolved grief may contribute to social phobia. She suggests that "a truly biopsychosocial integration might allow us to make use of each of the modalities at a given point in time when specific patients can use them, and thereby potentiate a fuller, more felicitous recovery with longevity" (p. 6).

Research findings indicate significant comorbidity rates among anxiety disorders, including social phobia. Julieta Montejo and Michael Liebowitz comprehensively review epidemiological and clinical studies, noting that comorbidity research on social phobia is "still in an early stage" (p. 20). They conclude that a common methodological framework is needed to facilitate fully reliable comorbidity studies.

David Barlow and his colleagues have conducted extensive research on and treatment of anxiety disorders using a cognitive-behavioral

Mr. Beard is managing editor of the *Bulletin of the Menninger Clinic,* The Menninger Clinic, Topeka, Kansas.

group therapy approach. Their findings suggest that social phobia is often accompanied by personality disorders, substance abuse, and other anxiety and mood disorders. Pending further research, Barlow suggests that "the best strategy at the current time is to treat social phobia directly if it presents as the principal diagnosis and to carefully observe the effects on comorbid conditions" (p. 52).

Evidence indicates a high rate of comorbidity between social phobia and alcohol abuse. John Marshall discusses possible reasons for this relationship, and then describes approaches to diagnosis and therapy in both alcohol treatment and mental health settings. He notes that while social phobia in patients in alcohol treatment settings is often overlooked, "the excessive use of alcohol so commonly found with social phobia is also often overlooked in settings that treat social phobia" (p. 60).

Although historically pharmacotherapy has not been considered a primary approach to social phobia, recent clinical trials and case reports suggest that psychotropic agents can provide effective treatment. Recognizing that the comorbidity of social phobia with other conditions poses special clinical challenges, Jerrold Rosenbaum and Rachel Pollock outline principles of pharmacotherapy and suggest that a flexible approach is the best strategy.

In the concluding paper, Walter Menninger acknowledges that past difficulty in recognizing social phobia and its frequent comorbidity with other psychiatric conditions combine to pose a particular treatment challenge. He highlights eight operating principles to guide clinicians toward effective, integrated treatment, noting that "for these conditions, any of several treatment options may be equally efficacious" (p. 86, 88).

Our distinguished panel of authors wrote these papers in preparation for a symposium presented at the 1994 annual meeting of the American Psychiatric Association in Philadelphia, Pennsylvania. Both the symposium and this publication are supported by an unrestricted educational grant from Roche Laboratories, a member of the Roche Group. We extend our sincere thanks to the faculty; to the staff of Triclinica Communications who provided invaluable logistical support; and to our sponsors at Roche Laboratories for making this project possible. Finally, we recognize the extensive assistance of Jon Allen, PhD, editor of the *Bulletin of the Menninger Clinic;* the clinicians who served as referees; and the professional editorial staff of the *Bulletin,* including Mary Ann Clifft, Eleanor Bell, and Sharon Edmonds.

1. Uncharted Waters: Psychodynamic Considerations in the Diagnosis and Treatment of Social Phobia

Kathryn J. Zerbe, MD

Her strength and her limitations were that she didn't really know how it felt to be someone else. What she did know was how it felt to be alone, unique, isolated. (Spender, 1920, p. 141)

It may be comfortably assumed that, when making any diagnosis, clinicians can only delineate and classify what they know. Understanding and mastering a disorder is predicated on first recognizing that it is an affliction and then attempting to allay suffering it has caused with available therapeutics. Social phobia, the "marked and persistent fear of one or more social or performance situations.... [that] almost invariably provokes anxiety" (American Psychiatric Association [APA], 1993, p. K:5), culminates in the avoidance of a host of feared social and performance situations. Yet it has only been studied in depth in American psychiatry since 1985 (Liebowitz, Gorman, Fyer, & Klein, 1985). In view of the substantial morbidity occasioned by this disorder, one might reasonably wonder why scrutiny into its classification, etiology, and treatment has been so sparse relative to other disorders outside the British Isles.*

Anecdotal comments by practicing psychiatrists and other mental health professionals who are asked about their experience in treating social phobia reveal that it may go unaccounted for because it is not recognized or regarded as a serious problem. Since social phobia achieved recognition as a bona fide psychiatric disorder only in *DSM-III* (APA, 1980), one might understand this frequently encountered disclaimer: "Social phobia—I really don't see it that often, if at all." In a series of 3,106 discharges from the adult hospital of the C.F. Menninger Memorial Hospital from 1989 through 1993, only 12 pa-

---

Dr. Zerbe is vice president for Education, Research, and Applications, The Menninger Clinic, Topeka, Kansas.
*The reported lifetime diagnosis of social phobia in the United States is 2-3%, although contemporary research reveals that this figure may be as high as 10% if the population is adequately diagnosed (Davidson, 1993). One study from the Maudsley Hospital in London found a full 8% of patients seeking treatment to be suffering from social phobia (Kleinknecht, 1992), but these investigators were highly attuned to the presentation of this disorder.

tients (fewer than 1%) carried a diagnosis of social phobia at discharge, and only one of these had a principal diagnosis of social phobia. Of 1,400 admissions to the Adult Outpatient Department of The Menninger Clinic, 45 patients (3%) were diagnosed with social phobia, with 17 (1%) carrying it as a principal diagnosis.

Should one assume that this diagnosis is really as uncommon or obscure as these observations imply? One could argue that these clinical samples are too small or unrepresentative. More accurate would be data derived from larger samples, rigorous population-based studies, semistructured interviews, and the like. Although these perspectives have clear merit and underscore the need for more research and systematic review of this condition, knowing what clinicians do or fail to do, based on the experience of actual practice parameters, is also important. We should assume that clinicians underdiagnose social phobia and wonder why (Montejo & Liebowitz, 1994).

These questions also have special relevance for psychiatric education, where primacy is placed on other recognizable and more established conditions such as schizophrenia, affective and personality disorders, and the eating disorders. Outside of specialized anxiety disorders clinics, do clinicians trained in this decade who will be practicing in the 21st century recognize this affliction that we summarize under the rubric of "fear of humiliation"? To assure accurate diagnosis and state-of-the-art treatment, formal didactic classes and concomitant clinical experience will need to be well intermeshed to ensure that this disorder is not a mere footnote in the curriculum of psychiatrists. These inferences also have implications for national health care policy, where radical assumptions are being made with regard to who can diagnose and treat psychiatric problems. The widening scope of practice for primary care providers now seems to include even mental disorders. Can one individual reasonably keep in mind so many facts and figures with respect to all the ills that befall humankind? If, for example, psychiatrists find the classification barrier between social phobia and avoidant personality somewhat murky, how will others with less finely tuned diagnostic skills be able to recognize and effectively intervene with a condition that all too frequently culminates in the abuse of alcohol and/or other substances, or even leads to suicide (Liebowitz, 1987; Marshall, 1994; Turner, Beidel, Dancu, & Keys, 1986)?

Considering the neglect of this subject by general psychiatry, it is also a puzzling, if not disconcerting, fact that contemporary psychoanalysis has also scotomized it. Classical psychoanalysis was launched on the tarmac of Freud's case study method, where different kinds of phobias were not only the presenting symptoms but also caused their victims to endure tremendous suffering (Appignanes & Forrester, 1992; Breuer & Freud, 1893-1895/1955; Gay, 1988; A. Freud, 1977; S. Freud, 1895/1962a, 1895/1962b). Despite the notable history of psychoanalysis in describing the toll that phobias take in an individual's life (often to the point of arresting psychological development and human potential altogether), it has paradoxically not brought forth a concomitant breadth of understanding and treatment possibilities for those sufferers. That is, with relatively few exceptions, the contemporary psychoanalytic literature is sparse with respect to the general theory of phobias and treatment applications (Compton, 1992a, 1992b; Gabbard, 1990, 1992, 1994; Kohut, 1984).

This perplexing and unfortunate state of affairs is particularly striking inasmuch as psychoanalysis owes a great debt to those early patients who—often with considerable shame and only by overcoming great stigma, even by modern standards—sought treatment. For example, a little over a century ago, Baroness Fanny Moser sought out the famous Viennese physician Josef Breuer, who then referred her to his protégé Sigmund Freud. Among her many complaints, which included clacking, grimaces, tics, fear of animals, preoccupation with death and loss, anorexia, and disgust and resentment at various family members, she told Freud that she had a "dread of strangers, and of people in general" (Breuer & Freud, 1893-1895/ 1955, p. 87). Freud's now-famous patient, to whom he gave the pseudonym Frau Emmy von N., may, by current diagnostic standards, be considered the first comprehensively described social phobia patient in the psychoanalytic literature.

A rereading of Frau Emmy von N.'s case history gleans that she fulfills many of the *DSM-IV* (APA, 1993) criteria for social phobia. Through the crevices of her amalgamation of complaints, we read that she grew to fear social situations in which she felt "exposed to unfamiliar people or to possible scrutiny by others" (criterion A), certain social situations provoked anxiety (criterion B) that did not abate, and she seemed to recognize that her fear was "excessive or unreasonable" (criterion C). That is to say, she had insight and was not delusional, although at times her symptomatology seemed to suggest what we would currently view as "lower level pathology" (i.e., borderline personality disorder). She readily accepted Freud's suggestion that she be housed in a nursing home for treatment, thereby fulfilling criterion D, the avoidance of "feared social or performance situations." However, Freud did not choose to focus on these particular symptoms. Like modern clinicians, his diagnostic and therapeutic punch drove straightaway into those difficulties that caused his patient her most unremitting symptoms, following the classification of symptoms he was then developing. Freud believed that Frau Emmy von N. was suffering from hysteria or, when actual traumatic experiences could be elucidated in the history, an *aktual* neurosis (Compton, 1992a, 1992b; Freud, 1895/1962a, 1895/1962b).

This famous psychoanalytic case history parallels what the current zeitgeist has to say about social phobia in still more fundamental ways. Just as a host of difficulties perplexed Frau Emmy von N. and her young, striving doctor, patients with social phobia complain of a plethora of other psychiatric problems that often take precedence in formal diagnostic reports and treatment planning. That is, social phobia is highly comorbid for other psychiatric disorders; the diagnosis may often be missed or go unnoted when other conditions are felt to be more prominent, preoccupying, or life threatening (Ross, 1993; Schneier, Johnson, Hornig, Liebowitz, & Weissman, 1992). Clinicians assume that no one ever dies of social phobia. But concern increases with respect to conditions that may lead to death, such as depression, anorexia nervosa, and alcoholism. Hence it is not surprising that social phobia has been "almost completely ignored by the health care system" (Ross, 1993, p. 5), even though current surveys suggest that more than 10% of the population may be afflicted by the seemingly unreasonable symptom of fear in social situations that leads to social avoidance (Davidson, 1993).

Countertransference issues

Attuning our psychotherapeutic ear to the question of why we so readily miss the diagnosis of social phobia, and consequently know relatively little about it, we may be given to ask: What gets in the way of our hearing our patients' symptoms about fear of social and performance situations? Perhaps the answer is at least partially imbedded in an unrecognized countertransference phenomenon. Who among us has not felt (even as we might wish to forget or deny it) intense anxiety about "feared social or performance situations" (criterion D) that we realize is "excessive or unreasonable" (criterion C) and endured the symptoms of a queasy stomach or a racing heart or sweaty palms (criterion B) in such a performance situation where one undergoes scrutiny by others (criterion A)? We miss diagnosing social phobia because we clinicians, like most people, have ourselves been beset by social anxiety at one time or the other. Usually, we get over it quickly enough so that it does not generalize (Liebowitz, 1987) or become an entrenched way of behaving (e.g., become a phobia). Yet our personal experience of having the feelings—but then getting over them—may lead us to lose empathy for our burdened patients (Jackson, 1992). A paradox of human nature is that we study hardest that which we most need to master (e.g., mastery by intellectualization and/or sublimation), while simultaneously emotionally distancing ourselves from peculiarities and quirks in others that we believe we have long since abandoned (e.g., defensive denial).

Naturally enough, we can rationalize our blind spots, arguing that social phobia is a relatively new disorder and that pinpointing it pales in comparison to the accurate assessment of someone who is floridly psychotic or suicidally depressed or in the midst of a fulminating panic attack. Yet the interference that social anxiety brings to a person's normal day can wreak havoc on occupational strivings and social relationships (criterion E). Social phobia is responsible for larger economic loss, greater interpersonal disruption, and deeper personal pain than can be easily measured by modern accounting methods. We do know that some of the costs include alcohol dependence, depression, agoraphobia, inability to form and maintain lasting relationships, and stymied career goals, to name only a few (Ross, 1993).

The sense of shame that clinicians feel when identifying with some of the symptoms of their patients with social anxiety, and the sense of hubris engendered by the feeling that one has overcome it, may indeed be the major countertransference pitfalls encountered in practice. Still another countertransference difficulty faced when making the diagnosis of social phobia is the uncertainty with which we approach treatment. Although all medical practitioners take solace in the fact that the Hippocratic oath admonishes us to "first, do no harm," in actuality we all want to "do something" and make our patients, in the words of the late Dr. Karl Menninger, "weller than well" (Menninger, Mayman, & Pruyser, 1963, p. 406). Although heartened by the recent outpouring of studies in the pharmacotherapy (Liebowitz, 1993; Marshall, 1992) and cognitive-behavioral literature (Barlow, 1992; Heimberg, 1993; Heimberg & Barlow, 1988; Kleinknecht, 1991) regarding social phobia, we practitioners struggle with the limits of our craft. Despite the favorable results of these modalities, neither treatment approach is a panacea. Sophisticated research studies demonstrate that the relapse rate is high following drug termination, that symptoms improve but are not totally ameliorated by cognitive-behavioral modalities, and that there remains a "need for the development of multiple and diverse alternatives for the treatment of social phobia" (Heimberg, 1993, p. 36). In particular, studies that assess the additive effects of the most useful medications and cognitive-behavioral interventions are sorely needed, as are studies that allow us to delineate which patients might best partake of particular interventions and strategies and for how long.

Forging a listening model

As a specialty, psychiatry is still in its infancy with respect to comprehending why some patients respond psychotherapeutically to cognitive-behavioral or psychodynamic interventions based on their own ways of knowing (Belenky, Clinchy, Goldberger, & Tarule, 1986) and understanding the world. Still in question is to what extent the practitioner or the technique itself effects change and to what degree each contributes to improvement. Likewise, more often than most would like to admit with respect to medication selection, we clinicians choose drugs based on our own idiosyncratic usage. More specific ways of delineating which drug fits which kind of patient, based on empirical data, must be identified and utilized. In the treatment of social phobia, psychopharmacological practice has shifted dramatically since the late 1980s, and it will likely continue to evolve rapidly. Thus the state of the art in treating social phobia at this juncture in psychiatric history is both a curious and mixed picture. Pharmacotherapy does well, but no one knows for certain how long, particularly once the drug is discontinued. Cognitive-behavioral interventions also do well, but no one knows exactly why or if they do as well as might be ideal. With both modalities leaving room for improvement, if not good argument, one would assume that there could be great opportunity for psychodynamically oriented theory (Zerbe, 1990) to add a helpful and unique perspective. When we turn to the psychoanalytic literature on the subject, we find a very thin selection of work. Perhaps the recognition that ultimate answers are still to be found regarding the treatment of social phobia will be most heartening to trainees who are looking for a subspecialty that has not yet been fully mined with respect to the most highly efficacious treatments and the rationale for their choice.

One might also speculate, however, that the understanding and treatment of social phobia could be one crucible for the coming together of *each* of the foregoing perspectives to more fully understand the inner biological workings and psychological contingencies of the patient (Menninger, 1992). That is, a truly biopsychosocial integration might allow us to make use of each of the modalities at a given point in time when specific patients can use them, and thereby potentiate a fuller, more felicitous recovery with longevity. In this regard, one could extend the question about what current psychoanalytic thinking might add to the treatment of patients with social phobia. In the remainder of this paper, I will describe two cases in which social phobia was a prominent aspect of the clinical course of a patient. This case material will enable us to explore some ways that contemporary psychoanalytic thought amplifies or sheds light on the patient's experience of social avoidance and seeks to enable that patient to overcome the anxiety of the feared performance situations by understanding, insight, ego strengthening, and a reduction in superego pressure.

Because the psychodynamic understanding of social phobia has garnered such little attention in the psychoanalytic literature, we have had to step aside from particular theories and traditions and instead attune our ears directly toward the cues provided by the patient. This approach best enables us to learn what is important, when, and why. Again, it will be demonstrated that the patient is always our best teacher if we can only lay down our theories long enough to hear. But in so doing, there is an excellent historical precedent: It was Frau Emmy von N. herself who bluntly gave Freud his most famous reprimand. Not satisfied by her doctor's use of hypnotic suggestions and admonitions to change her behavior, Frau Emmy forcefully told Freud to be quiet and to allow her to speak. He had apparently gotten in the way of her telling an all-too-human story of trauma and loss by resolutely holding on to his own technique. According to Freud, Frau Emmy tackled his tenacity about "asking her where this and that came from, but let her tell me what she had to say" (quoted in Gay, 1988, p. 70). By listening to this patient, Freud chanced upon the technique of free association, learned firsthand the limitations of the behavioral-hypnotic suggestions he was employing, and came smack up against a multitude of traumatic memories that had bedeviled Frau Emmy. Alas, despite her improvement with what Freud called "the cathartic procedure" (Breuer & Freud, 1893-1895/1955, p. 105), Frau Emmy's improvement was also not sustained.

Yesterday's inadequacies introduced the present puzzle. Glimpsed was the import of traumatic memories and incidents that begged for a nonjudgmental other in a safe space (e.g., Winnicott's [1965] holding environment) to mollify what was most powerfully enigmatic and stultifying to development. Left was the quagmire of what to do for persistent phobias and major life impairment, a stalemate that the biological therapies and cognitive sciences have done so much to reverse. However, because these methods are also imperfect and imprecise, clinicians may choose to draw on psychodynamic principles in their understanding and treatment of patients. We will not infrequently be surprised by how often human encounters with shame, trauma, and loss play major roles in the etiology of social phobia.

Show—Don't tell

In many cases of social phobia, shame is considered an important underlying dynamic (Gabbard, 1992); fear of public humiliation derives from an inner conviction of one's basic defectiveness, incompetence, and deficiency (Miller, 1985). Shame is a complex emotion whose underbelly may hide reaction formation (Miller, 1985), sexual anxieties (Broucek, 1991), conflicts over pride, competition, and dependency (Nathanson, 1992), narcissism (Broucek, 1991; Lewis, 1987; Nathanson, 1987; Wurmser, 1981, 1987), and struggles with aggression (Miller, 1985; Nathanson, 1992; Piers & Singer, 1953). Conflicts over aggression lead the patient to project a harsh superego outwardly onto those who might inflict punishment. Avoidance of social situations believed to be foolish and the accompanying disorganizing anxiety are driven by unmetabolized aggression as much as by lowered self-esteem and self-hatred. As Miller (1985) has further explicated with respect to shame, "One emphasizes the foolish side of one's actions rather than the aggressive aspect, because at one moment it is less threatening to see one's self as humiliated than to see one's self as hostile" (p. 132).

Shame is difficult to communicate (Lynd, 1958) to another human being, and one might reasonably wonder how each individual who experiences it struggles to begin to deal with it and put it in words. The clinician may silently have in mind this question when encountering the patient: What is shamed in the shaming experience? Shame makes one feel vulnerable and the object of scorn or ridicule from an audience. Patients with social phobia who struggle with underlying shame are terrified that others will come to know who they really are and that they will be found sorely lacking. By eschewing the feared performance situations in which they might fail, they avoid taking risks and encountering the potential ridicule and frustration that might be met should they fail.

In contrast, individuals more at peace with their own uniqueness realize that success and failure are part of every life. As one patient philosophically captured this daily struggle of worth, victory, and defeat, "Playing a sport helps me deal with life. Some days you go out and everything you do seems right. Other times, you are totally off base and clumsy. You lose. Life is like that with its ups and downs." This individual has developed a stable self-image, unperturbed by overwhelming narcissism, greed, hostility, selfishness, competition, and envy; he is not afraid to lose or to be made a fool—at least temporarily—because he realizes that this is the stock in trade of *all* human beings. He can discharge appropriate aggression and competition into a culturally sanctioned and social activity (e.g., sports). He has perspective. He can laugh at himself.

Not so for those individuals who wrestle mightily with shame. To protect themselves from even greater vulnerability and exposure, they avoid the situations they most fear by, metaphorically, "hiding their light under a bushel." Their behavior belies a deep lack of trust in others to accept them for their uniqueness—assets and liabilities alike. Consequently, a wide array of gratifying and challenging experiences are never undertaken; failures are also bypassed because they cannot risk failing. Fear of humiliation hinders these individuals from truly testing their wings while it precludes them from knowing the limits of their range.

Case example

Ms. A was the older child and only daughter in a sibship of two. Her scholarly engineer father scolded her for any grade less than an A, particularly in math. Her mother, a homemaker who held degrees in music and architecture, accepted her husband's terrifying outbursts with a cowering demeanor and self-sacrificial attitude. After any vicious fight between the two adults, the mother would then rage at her daughter for not doing more of the household chores, which she believed brought on her husband's wrath.

In psychoanalysis, the patient also recalled how her father never seemed pleased with her grades or with the amount of work or duties she performed. When she began to demonstrate some precocious abilities with essay writing and poetry to the point of winning some local literary contests, he needled her for her lack of interest in math and girls' athletics; he also demeaned her for her inability to beat him at pinochle or bridge. From the patient's perspective, she was faced with an insolvable dilemma. If she tried to win her father's approval by academic achievement based on her natural abilities, he rejected her. Unable and unwilling to fulfill his other dreams and aspirations, she retreated from the anger she felt out of fear of his retaliation. She felt that her mother was unavailable and unable to give comfort. Conflicts about performance were not limited to the family; the patient stayed as quiet as she could, never sharing her "secret" poetry with anyone until well into her third year of psychoanalysis.

At this juncture in the treatment, the patient received a request to read some of her poems when she accepted a national writing award. She was convinced that she would be exposed for what she considered her "lackluster productions," yet she recognized that her fears were totally unwarranted. Nevertheless, considering the public recognition implied by the award, she declined to speak. We then learned that her fear of performance in this situation dovetailed with other worries about general social situations. Dating provoked enormous anxiety. Although she never turned to alcohol to self-medicate, became seriously depressed, or exhibited suicidal ideation, her social phobia substantially interfered with her professional and social interactions. She was convinced that she could never "measure up" to the demands of other people—be it a boss, an audience, or a mate.

One can safely assume that the early traumatogenic environment of this patient played a substantial role in the etiology of her social phobia. Although a widening definition of trauma has been implicated in the etiology of other psychiatric disorders (e.g., bulimia nervosa [Zerbe, 1993]), a parental union rife with venomous verbal exchanges, and possibly even physical assaults, has not previously been suggested in the contemporary psychodynamic literature with respect to social phobia. This patient felt humiliated by both of her parents and frustrated in her attempts to please either of them. Such humiliation is often the key in the experience of shame when the child may also serve as a repository of the parents' projected feelings of shame and failure (Broucek, 1991). Concomitantly, the patient had to suppress, repress, and then displace her feelings of normal competition, pride, and anger, leading to a thwarting of her nascent sense of self. Expressing the forbidden would unleash abuse, hence her generalized fear should she "show herself" to another human being.

In the analysis, I came to know the patient's feelings of shame, humiliation, and social anxiety via projective identification. Any intervention I made was met by a comment that either negated my point in toto or, more subtly, criticized me for being slightly off the mark. I experienced firsthand her burden; she was hindered from social action by her parents' attacks and outbursts (Broucek, 1991). In this case, I found myself hesitating in making certain interventions and interpretations when otherwise I would have felt clearly capable of doing so, convinced as I was that the patient would counter my comments with a shame-provoking criticism or, more persistently, with no acknowledgment that I had even spoken a word and was heard. Self-analysis revealed that the patient had induced in me a temporary state of social phobia or fear of humiliation so that I hesitated to speak my mind to her devaluing, vigilant, angry internalized parental image.

Shame strips the individual of wanting to connect on an interpersonal level lest one encounter one's own nakedness in a most infelicitous environment. Social phobia, based on the dynamics of shame, humiliation, and unacknowledged anger, may also create a brief encounter with interpersonal avoidance in the therapist. Perhaps this avoidance also factors into the difficulty clinicians have in making the diagnosis of social phobia more often.

Reexamining this clinical vignette from the perspective of self psychology (Kohut, 1971, 1977, 1984, 1985) sheds further insight into the dynamics of social phobia. For this patient, the age-appropriate need to be mirrored and valued for her talents and for her own self were not met by either parent. Lacking affirmation, the patient began to fragment, leading to a host of psychiatric symptomatology. Her social phobia was not the initial reason for seeking treatment; like other patients, she entered analysis because she was chronically dysphoric, unable to achieve professionally to the degree she would like, and unhappy in her relationships. Only over the course of a prolonged treatment did all the symptoms become evident and the full recognition of their impact on her life become appreciated. Experiences that would normally produce joy when met with delight and approbation by parents had not been present in her family of origin. Instead, the patient was incessantly and mercilessly assailed. She became understandably alarmed at even the thought of allowing her gifts to come out from behind the shadows. Haughtily criticized by the paternal selfobject, she avoided public appearance and certain performance situations (criterion E). By the apprehensive, cowering responses of the maternal selfobject, the patient became overwhelmed and panicked when exposed to the feared social situation (criterion B).

The backdrop of parental conflict led the patient to be insecure with respect to ever finding a supportive partnership that would nurture her growth. Without the experience of a calming mother as a selfobject who would nurture self-soothing capacities to allay the spread of anxiety, the patient lacked the capacity to soothe herself. The structural defect that followed from her father's criticisms hindered the age-appropriate development of the grandiose sense of self, which would, with gradual but optimal failure, transform into attainable ambitions with the psychic structure to support them.

In retrospect, it appears that the father envied his child's developmental progress; her talents were a threat to his own cohesion. Without the benefit of adequate parental figures to support growth through transmuting internalization, patients are left with vulnerability to generalized anxiety (Zerbe, 1990), social phobia, and what they believe will be a likely public humiliation that they will not be able to endure or overcome. Such case histories suggest multigenerational failures of cohesion of the parent's self, while emphasizing the need for treaters to supply specific selfobject functions whether through the medium of medication or psychotherapy. One could further speculate that all therapeutic modalities currently used for treating social phobia converge to rectify these early selfobject failures by allaying anxiety and encouraging self-expression. Medication, cognitive-behavioral therapy, and more psychodynamically based psychotherapies all remedy "the deficiency of soothing" (Kohut, 1984, p. 215) and promote calmness so that the self may be strengthened to tackle feared situations.

Finally, reared in an environment utterly lacking in humor, the patient never developed the capacity to poke fun at herself, a powerful tool for reducing the pain of potential embarrassment or ridicule. Psychotherapeutic treatment should enable us to laugh "gently about some once-hidden subject, something that once caused searing pain" (Nathanson, 1992, p. 394). A sense of the comic helps to weather social anxieties because it reminds us of our own and others' foibles. We love ourselves and others best when we can make fun of the human tendency to take ourselves so seriously. As Nathanson (1992) also explained, "There is a laughter of love, a laughter that shows the sudden pleasure of self accompanying healthy new self-recognition" (p. 394).

The aftermath of loss

One does not commonly associate the development of phobia, particularly social phobia, with unresolved loss. The extant literature suggests that parental death may play a role, at least in the development of phobias in children, but no longitudinal case studies (Hummer, 1988) have pointed to a definitive connection. The work of Bowlby (1960, 1969, 1973, 1979a, 1979b, 1980) has demonstrated a host of difficulties that arise when children are traumatized by the loss of an affectional bond, including but not exclusively related to death. Adults, too, may react to grief productively or unproductively (Gut, 1989), using the affects of depression, helplessness, anger, loneliness, and anxiety as signals to push the organism toward repair.

Humans will most typically seek out other humans to share their most painful emotions and thereby interrupt or work through their responses to bereavement. If the individual has attained the capacity to trust others and is not ashamed of seeking help, bereavement may be a time when he or she seeks out another, particularly a treater, to ease the intensity of the pain. When the earliest relationship has been characterized as one of anxious attachment (Arbel & Stravynski, 1991; de Ruiter & van Ijzendoorn, 1992; West, Rose, & Sheldon, 1993), bereavement follows a different path. Anger, always hard to overtly express, may go underground as the person seeks another attachment figure in response to the pressure of abandonment anxiety. More often, the individual exhibits compulsive self-reliance (Parks, 1972), shunning the love and care of others that could be beneficial. These individuals often present to general practitioners with psychosomatic symptoms, depression, or phobias. Because individuals regard their phobias as strange and peculiar, they are less apt to share them. This may be particularly true for social phobia patients, for whom the very nature of their problem keeps them from seeking help (Kleinknecht, 1991). Hence the sample of psychosomatic illnesses and depression following grief may be inflated in comparison to an unusually small number of phobia patients who have difficulty sharing their difficulties.

Case example

Ms. B was a 29-year-old, unmarried, graduate student in business and public policy when she was referred for evaluation and possible psychotherapy. "Referred" is a clinical euphemism in this case. The patient was literally picked up and hauled off to the clinic by her neighbor, an esteemed clinical social worker, at the behest of the patient's ailing, widowed father. Ms. B's mother had died unexpectedly 6 months before the patient came for treatment. Subsequently, the patient found herself pervasively anxious in social situations, had difficulty using public restrooms, refused to attend seminars such that her future livelihood was in jeopardy, and could not contemplate making a public presentation of her work. She was most devoted and competent in caring for her ailing father. She was deeply ashamed that others believed she needed support and guidance to work through her loss.

Although the patient's history was replete with a variety of depressive and anxious symptoms present since her late teens, symptoms of social phobia appeared only subsequent to her mother's death. As she tortuously detailed her early life, the picture that emerged was of a latency age child and adolescent who had been anxiously attached to a very depressed, and possibly psychotic, mother. Other family members interviewed later in the treatment confirmed the sad history of a talented and giving mother who would periodically break down into fits of agitated depression and suicidality, often requiring hospitalization. The patient herself confided that she grew up always worrying about when her mother's next "breakdown" would occur. She suspected that she had to walk on tiptoe so as not to threaten the fragile equilibrium of her beloved mother, and she was both compliant with and subservient to her mother's needs.

Although the overt phobic symptoms interrupted the patient's occupational and social functioning, she refused all suggestions for medication. Preoccupied with a rash of murders that she had read about in another state, she became quite alarmed when the therapist announced an upcoming interruption. Calling from her home in a quite agitated state, she retorted that the therapist might really be Lynette "Squeaky" Fromme, the assailant of President Ford, even though she knew this idea was ridiculous. She responded to reassurance and the scheduling of another hour.

This case demonstrates several commonly touted dynamics about social phobia and illuminates some newer ones. First, the patient's development of a manifest anxiety disorder may have arisen due to exposure to one parent with a severe psychiatric disturbance. Gabbard (1994), in citing the work of Rosenbaum et al. (1992) and Kagan, Reznick, and Snidman (1988), explained that research supports the view that parents with a greater anlage of anxiety convey to their children a sense of dangerousness in the world, which may predispose them to phobias. This patient believed that she had "learned to be anxious" from watching her mother and had never developed a self-soothing capacity to sustain herself through life's exigencies, especially death. After her mother's death, Ms. B pathologically identified with some of her mother's symptomatology, remaining anxiety ridden and professionally compromised. The severe emotional trauma of her youth appears to have created within the patient a basic insecurity, so that she transferred "anxious attachment" to her father following her mother's death. Although one could surmise that she avoided heterosexual involvement as an oedipal defense against fantasied retaliation from the deceased mother, a more likely explanation in this case rests on her need to project her hostility and hatred for her mother onto the therapist. By assuming that the therapist was "Squeaky" Fromme and by staying socially incapacitated, the patient removed herself from the threat of her own aggressive impulses. By employing the defensive strategies of displacement, projection, and avoidance, the patient deployed the three defense mechanisms that most commonly signify phobic neurosis (Gabbard, 1994; Nemiah, 1981).

Most importantly, her social phobia developed as an apparent reaction to bereavement. Only within the context of intensive psychodynamically oriented therapy over many months was the patient able to acquire a self-soothing capacity and to work through her loss. Social phobia was the "vital process" (Gut, 1989) that led her to treatment for bereavement, not depression or complicated bereavement as might be expected. Turning a deaf ear to her personal pain by aggressive use of pharmacotherapy or behavioral techniques *may* have temporarily helped her phobia, but would not have touched its cause. If we clinicians maintain an open heart as well as an open mind, we will enable our patients to work through trauma, adapt to loss, and find satisfactory resolution to their existential pain. We will help make our patients' lives more bearable and, in the process, we may learn much more about the disorder we are attempting to study than if we stay bound and beholden to any *one* theory or treatment method.

References

American Psychiatric Association. (1980). *Diagnostic and statistical manual of mental disorders* (3rd ed.). Washington, DC: Author.

American Psychiatric Association. (1987). *Diagnostic and statistical manual of mental disorders* (3rd ed, rev.). Washington, DC: Author.

American Psychiatric Association. Task Force on DSM-IV. (1993). *DSM-IV draft criteria (3/1/93)*. Washington, DC: Author.

Appignanes, L., & Forrester, J. (1992). *Freud's women.* New York: Basic Books.

Arbel, N., & Stravynski, N.A. (1991). A retrospective study of separation in the development of adult avoidant personality disorder. *Acta Psychiatrica Scandinavica, 83,* 174-178.

Barlow, D.H. (1992). Cognitive-behavioral approaches to panic disorder and social phobia. *Bulletin of the Menninger Clinic, 56*(2, Suppl. A), A14-A28.

Belenky, M.F., Clinchy, B.M., Goldberger, N.R., & Tarule, J.M. (1986). *Women's ways of knowing: The development of self, voice, and mind.* New York: Basic Books.

Bowlby, J. (1960). Grief and mourning in infancy and early childhood. *Psychoanalytic Study of the Child, 15,* 9-52.

Bowlby, J. (1969). *Attachment and loss: Vol. I. Attachment.* New York: Basic Books.

Bowlby, J. (1973). *Attachment and loss: Vol. II. Separation: Anxiety and anger.* New York: Basic Books.

Bowlby, J. (1979a). *The making and breaking of affectional bonds.* London: Tavistock.

Bowlby, J. (1979b). On knowing what you are not supposed to know and feeling what you are not supposed to feel. *Canadian Journal of Psychiatry, 24,* 403-408.

Bowlby, J. (1980). *Attachment and loss: Vol. III. Loss: Sadness and depression.* London: Hogarth Press.

Breuer, J., & Freud, S. (1955). Studies on hysteria. In J. Strachey (Ed. and Trans.), *The standard edition of the complete psychological works of Sigmund Freud* (Vol. 2, pp. vii-xxxi, 1-311). London: Hogarth Press (Original work published 1893-1895)

Broucek, F.J. (1991). *Shame and the self.* New York: Guilford.

Compton, A. (1992a). The psychoanalytic view of phobias: I. Freud's theories of phobias and anxiety. *Psychoanalytic Quarterly, 61,* 206-229.

Compton, A. (1992b). The psychoanalytic view of phobias: II. Infantile phobias. *Psychoanalytic Quarterly, 61,* 230-253.

Davidson, J.R.T. (1993). Social phobia in review: 1993. *Journal of Clinical Psychiatry, 54*(12, Suppl.), 3-4.

de Ruiter, C., & van Ijzendoorn, M.H. (1992). Agoraphobia and anxious-ambivalent attachment: An integrative review. *Journal of Anxiety Disorders, 6,* 365-381.

Freud, A. (1977). Fears, anxieties, and phobic phenomena. *Psychoanalytic Study of the Child, 32,* 85-90.

Freud, S. (1962a). Obsessions and phobias. Their psychical mechanism and their aetiology. In J. Strachey (Ed. and Trans.), *The standard edition of the complete psychological works of Sigmund Freud* (Vol. 3, pp. 69-84). London: Hogarth Press (Original work published 1895)

Freud, S. (1962b). On the grounds for detaching a particular syndrome from neuraesthenia under the description "anxiety neurosis." In J. Strachey (Ed. and Trans.), *The standard edition of the complete psychological works of Sigmund Freud* (Vol. 3, pp. 85-117). London: Hogarth Press. (Original work published 1895)

Gabbard, G.O. (1990). *Psychodynamic psychiatry in clinical practice.* Washington, DC: American Psychiatric Press.

Gabbard, G.O. (1992). Psychodynamics of panic disorder and social phobia. *Bulletin of the Menninger Clinic, 56*(2, Suppl. A), A3-A13.

Gabbard, G.O. (1994). *Psychodynamic psychiatry in clinical practice: The DSM-IV edition.* Washington, DC: American Psychiatric Press.

Gay, P. (1988). *Freud: A life for our time.* New York: Norton.

Gut, E. (1989). *Productive and unproductive depression: Success or failure of a vital process.* New York: Basic Books.

Heimberg, R.G. (1993). Specific issues in the cognitive-behavioral treatment of social phobia. *Journal of Clinical Psychiatry, 54*(12, Suppl.), 36-45.

Heimberg, R.G., & Barlow, D.H. (1988). Psychosocial treatments for social phobia. *Psychosomatics, 29,* 27-37.

Hummer, K.M. (1988). Johnny: Mobilizing a child's capacity to mourn by means of psychotherapy. In S. Altschul (Ed.), *Childhood bereavement and its aftermath* (pp. 165-185). Madison, CT: International Universities Press.

Jackson, S.W. (1992). The listening healer in the history of psychological healing. *American Journal of Psychiatry, 149,* 1623-1632.

Kagan, J., Reznick, J.S., & Snidman, N. (1988). Biological bases of childhood shyness, *Science, 240,* 167-171.

Kleinknecht, R.A. (1991). *Mastering anxiety: The nature and treatment of anxious conditions.* New York: Insight Books/Plenum.

Kohut, H. (1971). *The analysis of the self: A systematic approach to the psychoanalytic treatment of narcissistic personality disorders.* New York: International Universities Press.

Kohut, H. (1977). *The restoration of the self.* New York: International Universities Press.

Kohut, H. (1984). *How does analysis cure?* (A. Goldberg, Ed.). Chicago: University of Chicago Press.

Kohut, H. (1985). On leadership. In H. Kohut, *Self psychology and the humanities: Reflections on a new psychoanalytic approach* (pp. 51-72). New York: Norton. (Original work written 1969-1970)

Lewis, H.B. (1987). Shame and the narcissistic personality. In D.L. Nathanson (Ed.), *The many faces of shame* (pp. 93-132). New York: Guilford.

Liebowitz, M.R. (1987). Social phobia. *Modern Problems in Pharmacopsychiatry, 22,* 141-173.

Liebowitz, M.R. (1993). Pharmacotherapy of social phobia. *Journal of Clinical Psychiatry, 54*(12, Suppl.), 31-35.

Liebowitz, M.R., Gorman, J.M., Fyer, A.J., & Klein, D.F. (1985). Social phobia: Review of a neglected anxiety disorder. *Archives of General Psychiatry, 42,* 729-736.

Lynd, H.M. (1958). *On shame and the search for identity.* New York: Harcourt, Brace.

Marshall, J.R. (1992). The psychopharmacology of social phobia. *Bulletin of the Menninger Clinic, 56*(2, Suppl. A), A42-A49.

Marshall, J.R. (1994). The diagnosis and treatment of social phobia and alcohol abuse. *Bulletin of the Menninger Clinic, 58*(2, Suppl. A), A58-A66.

Menninger, K., Mayman, M., & Pruyser, P. (1963). *The vital balance: The life process in mental health and illness.* New York: Viking.

Menninger, W.W. (1992). Integrated treatment of panic disorder and social phobia. *Bulletin of the Menninger Clinic, 56*(2, Suppl. A), A61-A70.

Miller, S. (1985). *The shame experience.* Hillsdale, NJ: Erlbaum.

Montejo, J., & Liebowitz, M.R. (1994). Social phobia: Anxiety disorder comorbidity. *Bulletin of the Menninger Clinic, 58*(2, Suppl. A), A21-A42.

Nathanson, D.L. (Ed.). (1987). *The many faces of shame.* New York: Guilford.

Nathanson, D.L. (1992). *Shame and pride: Affect, sex, and the birth of the self.* New York: Norton.

Nemiah, J.C. (1981). A psychoanalytic view of phobias. *American Journal of Psychoanalysis, 41,* 115-120.

Parkes, C.M. (1972). *Bereavement: Studies of grief in adult life.* New York: International Universities Press.

Piers, G., & Singer, M.B. (1953). *Shame and guilt: A psychoanalytic and a cultural study.* Springfield, IL: Charles C Thomas.

Rosenbaum, J.F., Biederman, J., Bolduc, E.A., Hirschfeld, D.R., Faraone, S.V., & Kagan, J. (1992). Comorbidity of parental anxiety disorders as risk for childhood-onset anxiety in inhibited children. *American Journal of Psychiatry, 149,* 475-481.

Ross, J. (1993). Social phobia: The consumer's perspective. *Journal of Clinical Psychiatry, 54*(12, Suppl.), 5-9.

Schneier, F.R., Johnson, J., Hornig, C.D., Liebowitz, M.R., & Weissman, M.M. (1992). Social phobia: Comorbidity and morbidity in an epidemiologic sample. *Archives of General Psychiatry, 49,* 282-288.

Spender, S. (1920). *World within world.* New York: Harcourt, Brace.

Turner, S.M., Beidel, D.C., Dancu, C.V., & Keys, D.J. (1986). Psychopathology of social phobia and comparison to avoidant personality disorder. *Journal of Abnormal Psychology, 95,* 389-394.

West, M., Rose, M.S., & Sheldon, A. (1993). Anxious attachment as a determinant of adult psychopathology. *Journal of Nervous and Mental Disease, 181,* 422-427.

Winnicott, D.W. (1965). *The maturational processes and the facilitating environment: Studies in the theory of emotional development.* New York: International Universities Press.

Wurmser, L. (1981). *The mask of shame.* Baltimore: Johns Hopkins University Press.

Wurmser, L. (1987). Shame: The veiled companion of narcissism. In D.L. Nathanson (Ed.), *The many faces of shame* (pp. 64-92). New York: Guilford.

Zerbe, K.J. (1990). Through the storm: Psychoanalytic theory in the psychotherapy of the anxiety disorders. *Bulletin of the Menninger Clinic, 54,* 171-183.

Zerbe, K.J. (1993). *The body betrayed: Women, eating disorders, and treatment.* Washington, DC: American Psychiatric Press.

2. Social Phobia: Anxiety Disorder Comorbidity

Julieta Montejo, MD
Michael R. Liebowitz, MD

The term "comorbidity," coined by Feinstein (1970), implies in the field of psychiatry the co-occurrence of two or more psychiatric disorders in the same individual within a defined period of time. Studies of comorbidity concern the frequency and interrelationship of the distinct disorders; both overlapping and distinct features are considered.

It has been only since the introduction of *DSM-III* (American Psychiatric Association [APA], 1980) that overlapping symptomatology of patients suffering from different anxiety disorders has been examined. One of the principal reasons that comorbidity of psychiatric disorders has not been extensively assessed until recently was the existence of hierarchical exclusionary rules present in diagnostic classification systems prior to *DSM-III-R* in 1987 (Brown & Barlow, 1992).

A comorbid diagnosis is of epidemiological and clinical importance, related not only to the course, outcome, and response to treatment, but also to diagnostic, etiological, and morbidity issues. In the Epidemiologic Catchment Area (ECA) study (Robins, Locke, & Regier, 1991), more than 60% of the respondents with at least one lifetime psychiatric disorder had two or more disorders. A recent study (Kessler et al., 1994) of lifetime and 12-month prevalence of *DSM-III-R* psychiatric disorders in the United States found an even higher rate of comorbidity, affecting 79% of the respondents.

Comorbidity can be studied in several ways: either cross-sectionally or longitudinally; either in clinical or epidemiological samples; with different diagnostic systems and, accordingly, different instruments of assessment; and with various thresholds for considering diagnostic entities. Although necessary, there are still no generally established rules to evaluate comorbidity. This explains the differing interpretations of the issue and also the sometimes conflicting available data.

There are at least four uses of the primary-secondary diagnostic distinction: the first three are: (1) chronological, primary diagnosis (the first diagnosis temporally); (2) causal, secondary diagnosis (caused by another preexisting disorder); and (3) symptomatic predominance (the primary diagnosis is associated with the greatest dis-

Dr. Montejo is a staff psychiatrist at the Hospitale de la Princesa, Universidad Autónoma, Madrid, Spain. At the time this article was written, she was a visiting psychiatrist at the New York State Psychiatric Institute, New York City, where Dr. Liebowitz is director of the Anxiety Disorders Clinic.

tress or life interference) (Barlow, DiNardo, Vermilyea, Vermilyea, & Blanchard, 1986; Klerman, 1990). The fourth use, as established in *DSM-III-R,* describes the "principal" diagnosis as the condition that is chiefly responsible for occasioning the evaluation or admission and that may be the focus of attention or treatment. In each condition, comorbidity patterns will represent different issues, depending on which primary-secondary diagnostic distinction is made.

A study by de Ruiter, Rijken, Garssen, van Schaik, and Kraaimaat (1989) of comorbidity among anxiety disorders clearly demonstrated that investigation of comorbidity produced different findings, depending on which procedure was conducted for assessing comorbidity. Agreeing with them, we believe it is best for treatment planning to assign the principal diagnosis on the basis of degree of impairment. It will then be necessary to describe the temporal relationship between the disorders because, as de Ruiter et al. pointed out, a temporal viewpoint may provide insight into the etiology of the disorders. With this approach, secondary or additional comorbid disorders may be chronologically primary, secondary, or concomitant in onset with the principal disorder.

Social phobia: Anxiety disorder comorbidity

Research on anxiety disorders shows significant comorbidity rates, both between the various anxiety conditions and with other psychiatric and medical disorders. Social phobia is no exception. However, although other anxiety disorders have become the subject of increasing investigation, social phobia remained relatively unstudied until 1985 (Liebowitz, Gorman, Fyer, & Klein, 1985). Comorbidity research on social phobia is therefore still in an early stage.

There are some relevant epidemiological and clinical studies of social phobia comorbidity among anxiety disorders (see Table 1). In many cases, social phobia is considered a secondary disorder, while in others it is considered the primary disorder. There are also cases in which it is difficult to determine the primary diagnosis.

Epidemiological studies
Wittchen, Essau, and Krieg (1991) studied the similarities and differences in comorbidity in anxiety disorders, both in epidemiological and clinical samples. They reported that comorbidity rates within anxiety disorders were particularly high in the clinical sample and less so in the epidemiological group, but they did not evaluate social phobia.

Schneier, Johnson, Hornig, Liebowitz, and Weissman (1992) studied social phobia comorbidity in more than 13,000 adults from four U.S. communities involved in the ECA study. Agoraphobia, simple phobia, and obsessive-compulsive disorder were the anxiety disorders with the highest rate of co-occurrence with social phobia. In terms of lifetime rate per 100 persons, social phobia was comorbid with simple phobia 59% of the time; agoraphobia, 44%; obsessive-compulsive disorder, 11.1%; and panic disorder, 4.7%. The high rate of comorbidity of social phobia and agoraphobia may be explained

Table 1. *Comorbidity among social phobia (SP), agoraphobia (AGP), and panic disorder (PD)*

	Primary Diagnosis						
	Social Phobia			Agoraphobia		Panic Disorder	
Investigator	N	%AGP	%PD	N	%SP	N	%SP
Clinical samples							
Barlow et al., 1986	19	0	0	41	17	17	35
Solyom et al., 1986	47	30[a]	NR	80	55[b]	NR	–
Sanderson et al., 1987[c]	?	?	?	?	28	?	?
de Ruiter et al., 1989							
Interference procedure[d]	3	0	33	56[e]	11	17	6
Temporal procedure[f]	5	60	0	27[e]	0	10	0
Stein et al., 1989	NA	–	–	–	–	35[g]	46
DiNardo et al., 1990	48	2[e]	2	86[e]	9	67	16
Sanderson et al., 1990	24	NA	17[e]	NA	NA	55[e]	22
Van Ameringen et al., 1991	57	7	49.1[h]	NA	–	–	–
Starcevic et al., 1992	NA	–	35[e]	48	–	19	26.3
Andersch & Hanson, 1993	NA	–	–	NA	–	123[h]	26
Nonclinical samples							
Schneier, Johnson, et al., 1992	361	44.9	4.7	NA	–	–	–
Davidson et al., 1993	123	45.0	11.6	NA	–	–	–
Degonda & Angst, 1993	46[i]	43	34.7	44[j]	45	–	–

NA = not assessed; NR = not reported
[a]"Clinically significant agoraphobia"
[b]"Clinically significant social phobia"
[c]Summarized in Turner and Beidel (1989)
[d]Primary diagnosis based on degree of functional impairment
[e]Panic disorder with agoraphobia
[f]Primary diagnosis based on first syndrome to develop
[g]66% met criteria for agoraphobia
[h]Panic disorder with or without agoraphobia
[i]Social phobia with and without agoraphobia
[j]Agoraphobia with and without social phobia

in part by the overassignment of agoraphobia as a diagnosis in epidemiological studies (Horwath, Lish, Johnson, Hornig, & Weissman, 1993). Agoraphobia without panic disorder was thought common in the ECA studies, but in clinical rediagnosis many of these persons proved to have simple phobia. For subjects with comorbid disorders (except for agoraphobia, simple phobia, or schizophrenia, for which data are not available), social phobia preceded the comorbid disorder in 76.8% of cases, and had onset in the same year in 7.2% of cases. Only 31% of subjects with social phobia had no other lifetime disorder. Other anxiety disorders were the most common comorbid condition.

Degonda and Angst (1993) found a high rate of co-occurrence between agoraphobia and social phobia. Forty-five percent of all agoraphobia patients and 43% of all social phobia patients received both diagnoses over the 10-year period of the study.

Davidson, Hughes, George, and Blazer (1993) recently analyzed the epidemiology of social phobia based on findings from the Duke ECA study. They reported that the highest risk of a comorbid lifetime anxiety disorder in social phobia was simple phobia (60.8%), followed by agoraphobia (45.0%). (As mentioned previously, the apparent high risk for agoraphobia can be explained by an overdiagnosis of agoraphobia in the ECA studies.) The risk of panic disorder was 11.6%.

Epidemiological data (Beidel, 1991) indicate that anxiety disorders are the most common childhood disorder and that the comorbidity rate is high. Although Beidel's study does not provide specific rates of comorbidity among anxiety disorders, the results do indicate that children with social phobia could be differentiated by self-report inventories, daily diary data, and a psychophysiological assessment. These findings are important because they may suggest a way to recognize social phobia and prevent the full development of complications.

Clinical studies
Barlow et al. (1986) found that anxiety states almost always have additional diagnoses, whereas additional diagnoses occur less frequently with phobic disorders. In cases where panic disorder was the predominant clinical condition, comorbidity occurred 88% of the time and the majority of the additional diagnoses were social or simple phobias. When social phobia was the primary disorder, comorbidity occurred 47% of the time. Obsessive-compulsive disorder was comorbid in 10% of social phobia cases, while comorbidity with agoraphobia and panic disorder did not occur. In contrast, Solyom, Ledwidge, and Solyom (1986) reported that among social

phobia patients, 30% had clinically significant agoraphobia, and among agoraphobia patients, 55% had clinically significant social phobia.

Stein, Shea, and Uhde (1989) found that 46% of a sample of panic disorder patients had concomitant social phobia. Of this subgroup, 69% would have met the criteria for social phobia before the onset of panic disorder.

De Ruiter et al. (1989) reported that comorbidity among anxiety disorders was rather high and that social phobia was associated with one or more additional anxiety disorders in 67% of the sample. Their study used two definitions of what constitutes the primary diagnosis. When the criterion for a primary diagnosis was which disorder interfered most, panic disorder and agoraphobia were the primary diagnoses, but when the criterion was which came first, social and simple phobia were usually primary.

Among anxiety disorders, Sanderson, DiNardo, Rapee, and Barlow (1990) found an overall comorbidity rate of 70%. The comorbidity rate for social phobia was 58%. Simple phobia was comorbid with social phobia in 25% of cases; panic disorder with agoraphobia was comorbid with social phobia in 17% of cases.

A large majority (70.2%) of the social phobia patients studied by Van Ameringen, Mancini, Styan, and Donison (1991) suffered from at least one other anxiety disorder in their lifetime, in particular, panic disorder with or without agoraphobia (49.1%). Social phobia preceded the onset of panic disorder 60.7% of the time, and the onset of any other anxiety disorder 62.7% of the time.

In a study of comorbidity patterns of panic disorder and agoraphobia, Starcevic, Uhlenhuth, Kellner, and Pathak (1992) noted a high comorbidity rate of social phobia and panic disorder with agoraphobia (48%), compared to comorbidity of social phobia and panic disorder without agoraphobia (26.3%). They commented that the high comorbidity rate of social phobia and panic disorder with agoraphobia may also reflect the hypothesized role of social phobia and social-evaluation anxiety in predisposing panic disorder patients to develop agoraphobia (Pollard & Cox, 1988; Telch, Brouillard, Telch, Agras, & Taylor, 1989). Reinforcing this view, Scheibe and Albus (1992) pointed out that whereas patients with panic disorder without agoraphobia frequently exhibit no other anxiety disorder, patients with panic disorder with agoraphobia frequently suffer from additional anxiety disorders. In a sample of 123 panic disorder patients, Andersch and Hanson (1993) reported a prevalence of social phobia of 26%. Sixty-six percent of the patients had social phobia before the onset of panic disorder. The researchers found that agoraphobia was more frequent in panic disorder patients with concomitant social phobia (91%) than in those without social phobia (69%), and they concluded that concomitant social phobia in patients with panic disorder could be a marker for a more severe psychiatric illness.

Comorbidity patterns of social phobia and panic disorder with agoraphobia

As mentioned earlier, different rates of comorbidity between social phobia, panic disorder, and agoraphobia are found, depending on whether epidemiological or clinic studies are evaluated, and on what diagnostic system is used. Resulting rates vary widely, making the extent of comorbidity uncertain. Nonetheless, the co-occurrence of social phobia and agoraphobia and/or panic disorder seems high. We can therefore conclude that: (1) social phobia has a high rate of comorbidity with other anxiety disorders, (2) social phobia frequently precedes the onset of the comorbid condition, and (3) it is possible that preexisting social phobia influences the development of agoraphobia as a consequence of panic disorder. When social phobia and panic disorder co-occur, panic disorder is usually the more clinically troubling condition. This may be a consequence of age of onset. Because social phobia usually begins first, if it brings the patient to treatment, panic disorder comorbidity may not be present. When patients with social phobia and panic disorder do enter treatment, however, it is usually the more recent-onset panic disorder that has precipitated their search for medical attention. This would explain why panic disorder and agoraphobia comorbidity with social phobia are higher when panic disorder and agoraphobia are the primary disorders.

Agoraphobia and simple phobia seem to have the highest rate of comorbidity with social phobia in epidemiological samples (Davidson et al., 1993; Degonda & Angst, 1993; Schneier, Johnson, et al., 1992). Panic disorder, with or without agoraphobia, has higher rates in clinical samples (de Ruiter et al., 1989; Van Ameringen, Mancini, Styan, et al., 1991). Part of this may be explained by the overdiagnosis of agoraphobia without panic disorder in epidemiological studies (Horwath et al., 1993). It is also important to note that simple phobia and social phobia are the most frequent additional diagnoses when another anxiety disorder is the principal diagnosis (Barlow et al., 1986; de Ruiter et al., 1989; DiNardo & Barlow, 1990; Sanderson et al., 1990).

The high rates of comorbidity associated with anxiety disorders in general and social phobia in particular may be understood in terms of

Klein's (1991) "symptom progression model," as Wittchen et al. (1991) pointed out. Comorbidity may occur as part of the natural history of anxiety disorders. The following models are possible explanations of comorbidity: (1) persons inherit a vulnerability to anxiety per se and any disorder that develops may in fact be environmentally determined; (2) persons inherit a vulnerability to a specific anxiety disorder, which places them at risk for other anxiety disorders; and (3) persons inherit a vulnerability to several anxiety disorders, which unfold at specific, preprogrammed points in the life cycle. In the second model, treatment of social phobia should decrease the affected person's chances of developing other anxiety disorders, whereas this is less likely in the third model.

Primary social phobia encompasses three possible circumstances with regard to panic disorder and agoraphobia: (1) The patient suffers social phobia without any panic attacks; (2) the patient suffers social phobia as well as situation-bound panic attacks in social, interpersonal, or performance situations (probably the most common psychopathological circumstance); or (3) the patient suffers not only situational, stimulus-bound panic attacks, but also spontaneous panic attacks (i.e., the patient has *DSM-III-R* panic disorder). Patients who suffer from social phobia and spontaneous panic attacks may or may not develop agoraphobia or increased social avoidance. However, they may be at a higher risk for major depression (Stein et al., 1989).

Secondary social phobia represents the clinical course of some panic disorder patients in whom the fear of suffering panic attacks extends to the fear of embarrassment or humiliation were they to have a panic attack while around other people. Thus they avoid such activities as giving speeches and having parties. This secondary social phobia is not accorded independent diagnostic status in *DSM-IV*. However, if the unexpected panic attacks resolve and the social anxiety and avoidance persist, social phobia may merit such status, despite its historical evolution as a complication of panic disorder. In this regard, *DSM-IV* accords greater weight to the cross-sectional picture than did *DSM-III-R*.

Boundaries

The boundaries between social phobia, panic disorder, and agoraphobia have proven to be more difficult to articulate than expected. However, a review of the relevant literature suggests that social phobia is a specific diagnostic category that differs from panic disorder and agoraphobia on a number of variables.

Prevalence

Although previously both general population and clinical sample data have suggested that agoraphobia is more prevalent than social phobia, and that the rates of social phobia and panic disorder are comparable, a recent epidemiological study (Kessler et al., 1994) indicated that social phobia is the most common anxiety disorder, with a lifetime prevalence of 13% and a 12-month prevalence close to 8%. The lifetime prevalence rates of panic disorder and agoraphobia are 3.5% and 5.3%, respectively; 12-month prevalence rates are 2.3% and almost 3%, respectively (see Table 2).

Sociodemographic data

Social phobia appears to be equally common (48-60%) across genders in the majority of the clinical studies (Amies, Gelder, & Shaw, 1983; Andersch & Hanson, 1993; de Ruiter et al., 1989; DiNardo & Barlow, 1990; Sanderson et al., 1990; Solyom et al., 1986; Uhde, Tancer, Black, & Brown, 1991), although some studies (e.g., Gelernter, Stein, Tancer, & Uhde, 1992) have found social phobia to be more common in females (see Table 3). Agoraphobia is much more common in females, both in clinic subjects and in the general population. According to Kessler et al. (1994), the lifetime gender prevalence is 3.5% for males and 7.0% for females. Panic disorder is also more common in females both in clinical (Barlow et al., 1985) and epidemiological samples; again, Kessler et al.'s (1994) lifetime gender prevalence is 2.0% for males and 5.0% for females (see Table 3). In epidemiological studies, social phobia is more common in females (Davidson et al., 1993; Degonda & Angst, 1993; Schneier, Johnson, et al., 1992); Kessler et al. (1994) reported a lifetime gender prevalence of 11.1% for males and 15.5% for females.

Higher socioeconomic classes are overrepresented among social phobia clinical patients, whereas lower socioeconomic classes are predominant among epidemiological patients (Davidson et al., 1993; Eaton, Dryman, & Weissman, 1991; Schneier, Johnson, et al., 1992). Male social phobia patients, who generally have a better education level and a higher socioeconomic status, may be more likely to report impairment in functioning and thus may be more likely to seek treatment (Schneier, Johnson, et al., 1992). This could explain the lack of a gender difference and the reported higher socioeconomic status in clinical studies. In the Zurich epidemiological study (Degonda & Angst, 1993), there was no difference between subjects with any phobia and controls with regard to social class or level of education.

Social phobia seems to have an earlier age of onset than panic disorder and agoraphobia. As in clinical samples, social phobia in the

Table 2. *Lifetime prevalence (%) rates of social phobia, agoraphobia, and panic disorder*

Nature of Sample/ Investigator	Total N	Social Phobia	Agoraphobia	Panic Disorder
Clinical samples				
Marks, 1970	800[a]	8	60	NR
DiNardo et al., 1983	51[b]	16	45	16
Barlow, 1985	102[b]	19	40	17
Wittchen et al., 1991	101	NA	43.56	35.64
Nonclinical samples				
Myers et al., 1984[c]				
New Haven	3,058	NA	2.8	0.6
Baltimore	3,481	2.2	5.8	1.0
St. Louis	3,004	1.2	2.7	0.9
Pollard & Henderson, 1987, 1988				
Full *DSM-III* criteria	500	2.0	2.8	NA
Minus distress criterion	500	20.6	–	NA
Wittchen et al., 1991	133	NA	5.74	2.39
Eaton et al., 1991	14,400	2.73	5.63[d]	1.57[e]
Schneier, Johnson, et al., 1992				
Baltimore	3,481	3.1	NA	–
St. Louis	3,004	1.9	NA	–
Durham	3,921	3.2	NA	–
Los Angeles	3,131	1.8	NA	–
Davidson et al., 1993	3,801	3.8	NA	–
Degonda & Angst, 1993	591	5.4[f]	4.5[g]	NA
Kessler et al., 1994	8,098	13.3	5.3	3.5

NA = not assessed; NR = not reported
[a]Total phobia patients seen at Maudsley Hospital "in the last decade"
[b]Consecutive referrals to an anxiety clinic who were given a primary anxiety disorder diagnosis
[c]6-month prevalence rates
[d]Sample size for agoraphobia N = 14,436
[e]Sample size for panic disorder N = 19,501
[f]Lifetime prevalence of social phobia with and without agoraphobia
[g]Lifetime prevalence of agoraphobia with and without social phobia

community had a mean age of onset in the teenage years and was associated with a lower rate of marriage compared with the general population (Schneier, Johnson, et al., 1992). Onset of agoraphobia is generally between ages 20 and 30, while panic disorder usually appears to occur in the late 20s to early 30s (Burke, Burke, Regier, & Rae, 1990) (see Table 4).

Table 3. *Gender ratio of social phobia, agoraphobia, and panic disorder*

Nature of Sample/ Investigator	Social Phobia		Agoraphobia		Panic Disorder	
	N	%Female	N	%Female	N	%Female
Clinical samples						
Marks, 1970	64	50	480	75	NR	–
Amies et al., 1983	87	40	57	86	NA	–
Thyer et al., 1985	42	52	95	80	62	57
Solyom et al., 1986	47	47	80	86	NR	–
Sanderson et al., 1990	24	58	NA	–	55[a]	78
DiNardo et al., 1990	48	41	86[a]	82	67	67
Gelernter et al., 1992	66	64	NA	–	60[b]	62
Starcevic et al., 1992	NA	–	35[a]	57	19	52.6
Andersch & Hanson, 1993	32[c]	59	NA	–	91	63
Nonclinical samples						
Myers et al., 1984						
New Haven	NA	–	88	84	20	80
Baltimore	78	72	213	79	37	70
St. Louis	38	71	88	87	26	69
Pollard & Henderson, 1987, 1988						
Full *DSM-III* criteria	10	40	14	57	NA	–
Minus distress criterion	103	67	–	–	NA	–
Eaton et al., 1991	393	60	812	79	306	76
Schneier, Johnson, et al., 1992	361	69.5	NA	–	–	–
Davidson et al., 1993	123	62.7	NA	–	–	–
Degonda & Angst, 1993	46	69	44	66	NA	–
Kessler et al., 1994	1,077	59	429	67	283	72

NA = not assessed; NR = not reported
[a]Panic disorder with agoraphobia
[b]Panic disorder with and without agoraphobia
[c]Social phobia with panic disorder

Family studies

Some studies suggest that the relatives of panic disorder and agoraphobia patients are not at an increased risk for social phobia, nor are relatives of social phobia patients at an increased risk for panic disorder or agoraphobia (Mannuzza, Fyer, Liebowitz, & Klein, 1990). However, available data suggest that there is a familial contribution to the development of social phobia, although, as Fyer (1993) noted, only three studies have specifically addressed the heritability of social phobia. A family history study by Reich and Yates (1988) found increased rates of social phobia among the relatives of social phobia probands (6.6%), compared to relatives of panic disorder (0.4%) and normal control (2.2%) probands. A study by Kendler, Neale, Kessler, Heath, and Eaves (1992) of a sample of female twin pairs found that concordance for social phobia was greater for monozygotic (24%) than for dizygotic twins (15%), suggesting a genetic contribution. In a blind, controlled direct-interview family study of social phobia, Fyer, Mannuzza, Chapman, Liebowitz, and Klein (1993) found that relatives of social phobia probands had a significantly increased risk for social phobia (16%), compared to relatives of not ill controls (5%). Fyer et al. (1993) also concluded that there may be a heritable and partially genetic contribution to social anxiety and social phobia, although important contributions from nongenetic and otherwise nonheritable factors are also indicated. The authors noted that these initial findings require replication.

Biological studies

Biological challenge studies suggest that there may be differences in the underlying pathophysiology of social phobia and panic disorder. Sodium lactate infusion has demonstrated specificity in promoting panic attacks in panic disorder patients that do not seem to occur in

Table 4. *Ages of onset of social phobia and agoraphobia*

Investigator	Social Phobia		Agoraphobia	
	N	Mean age of onset	N	Mean age of onset
Marks & Gelder, 1966	25	18.9	84	23.9
Marks & Herst, 1970	NA	–	1,200	29.0
Shafar, 1976	20	20.0	68	32.0
Burns & Thorpe, 1977	NA	–	963	28.0
Sheehan et al., 1981	NA	–	100	24.1
Doctor, 1982	NA	–	404	28.1
Amies et al., 1983	87	19.0	57	24.0
Thyer et al., 1985	42	15.7	95	26.3
Cameron et al., 1986	37	14.3	NR	–
Turner et al., 1986	21	16.5	NA	–
Solyom et al., 1986	47		80	
First symptoms	–	16.6	–	24.5
Disorder	–	23.5	–	26.0
Ost, 1987	80	16.3	100	27.7
Van Ameringen et al., 1991	57	13.4	NA	–
Schneier, Johnson, et al., 1992	97	15.5	NA	–
Davidson et al., 1993	123	14.6	NA	–
Degonda & Angst, 1993	26	16.6	24	14.6

NA = not assessed; NR = not reported

social phobia patients. In one study (Liebowitz, Fyer, et al., 1985), only 7% of social phobia patients (vs. 44% of agoraphobia patients and 50% of panic disorder patients) experienced panic attacks when infused with 0.5 molar sodium lactate. In a study of carbon dioxide inhalation, administration of 5% CO_2 produced panic attacks in 39% of panic disorder and agoraphobia patients, in 8% of the control group, and in none of the patients with social phobia (Gorman et al., 1988).

Caffeine may induce panic attacks in social phobia patients at a rate comparable to that induced in panic disorder patients, although patients with social phobia have less severe anxiogenic responses and significantly lower rises in lactate after caffeine compared to patients with panic disorder. This suggests that the anxiety caused by caffeine may be related to baseline anxiety levels rather than to a specific diagnosis of social phobia (Tancer, 1993).

Following Uhde et al. (1991), we conclude that, compared to normal controls, panic disorder patients show a greater behavioral sensitivity to a wide variety of panicogens, including lactate, yohimbine, CO_2 inhalation, cholecystokinin, and isoproterenol. In contrast, social phobia patients have a relatively normal sensitivity to lactate, and they respond less severely to caffeine and CO_2 when compared with panic disorder patients.

Pharmacotherapy studies
Only a few placebo-controlled pharmacotherapy studies of social phobia have been conducted, but findings thus far indicate that monoamine oxidase inhibitors (MAOIs) and clonazepam are effective in the treatment of social phobia, although with high-potency benzodiazepines such as alprazolam and clonazepam a high rate of relapse may be seen following discontinuation (Liebowitz, 1993). These medications are also effective in panic disorder (Sheehan, Ballenger, & Jacobsen, 1980; Tesar et al., 1991). Tricyclic antidepressants do not appear to be efficacious in treating social discomfort in general or social phobia in particular (Liebowitz, 1987), while they are highly effective for panic disorder (Klein, 1964).

Phenelzine has proven to be significantly superior to both atenolol and placebo in treating social phobia (Liebowitz et al., 1992), and panic disorder (Sheehan et al., 1980) and social phobia both respond extremely well to this drug. Open trials have found fluoxetine effective for treating social phobia (Black, Uhde, & Tancer, 1992; Schneier, Chin, Hollander, & Liebowitz, 1992; Van Ameringen, Mancini, & Streiner, 1993) and panic disorder (Gorman et al., 1987; Schneier et al., 1990). Panic disorder patients (but not social phobia patients) show hypersensitivity to fluoxetine when initiating treatment, and they require very low starting doses (Gorman et al., 1987). Controlled studies are needed to evaluate fluoxetine's full treatment potential for both social phobia and panic disorder patients.

Beta-blockers do not reduce spontaneous panic attacks (Noyes et al., 1984), nor does pretreatment with beta-blockers prevent lactate-induced panic attacks in panic disorder patients (Gorman et al., 1983). However, beta-blockers appear successful in the acute reduction of certain aspects of performance anxiety (Liebowitz et al., 1985).

In a recent case report, Bakish (1994) found that brofaromine, a reversible specific MAO-A inhibitor, was helpful in the treatment of panic disorder with comorbid social phobia. Bakish also reported that fluoxetine helped reduce panic but not social phobia symptoms in a patient with both conditions.

Sleep studies

Sleep physiology is different for social phobia and panic disorder patients. The subjective and EEG sleep patterns of patients with social phobia are normal, whereas patients with panic disorder report a high lifetime rate of insomnia and sleep panic attacks. Sleep panic, which occurs during non-REM phases, may lead to the development of sleep phobias and chronic sleep deprivation in patients with panic disorder. Such sleep disruption may, in turn, induce an increased rate of panic attacks (Uhde et al., 1991).

Symptomatology

Regarding symptomatology, it is important to highlight that social phobia patients and panic disorder patients may experience different types of anxiety attacks (Mannuzza et al., 1990). The Schedule for Affective Disorders and Schizophrenia-Lifetime Anxiety Version (Mannuzza, Fyer, Klein, & Endicott, 1986) distinguishes three types of panic attacks: "spontaneous, out of the blue," "situationally predisposed," and "stimulus bound." Panic disorder is not simply characterized by having a panic attack, but rather as showing a recurrent pattern of attacks, at least some of which are spontaneous (Mannuzza et al., 1990).

According to *DSM-III-R* (APA, 1987), in social phobia "exposure to the specific phobic stimulus (or stimuli) almost invariably provokes an immediate anxiety response" (p. 243). As some authors note, the anxiety response of social phobia seems to be gradual rather than immediate. Nonetheless, this anxiety reaction may be experienced as subjective (e.g., distress, apprehensiveness, or discomfort), somatic (e.g., trembling, sweating, or palpitations), a combination of these responses, or a full-blown panic attack (Mannuzza et al., 1990).

When panic attacks occur in social phobia, they are generally associated with the phobic situation (mostly "stimulus bound") (Mannuzza et al., 1990); but when social phobia (either primary or secondary) is comorbid with panic disorder, "spontaneous" panic attacks occur. Barlow et al. (1985) found that only a minority of the panic attacks experienced by their simple phobia and social phobia patients were spontaneous.

Anxiety symptoms of social phobia and panic/agoraphobia appear to differ. Dizziness, difficulty breathing, weakness in limbs, fainting episodes, and buzzing or ringing in the ears are more common in agoraphobia patients, while blushing and muscle twitching are more common in social phobia patients (Amies et al., 1983). As Turner and Beidel (1989) reported, Gorman and Gorman (1987) also noted the presence of a specific subset of autonomic symptoms that seem particularly characteristic of social phobia patients: palpitations, trembling, sweating, and blushing.

A study by Reich, Noyes, and Yates (1988) also confirmed differences between anxiety symptoms in social phobia patients and panic disorder patients. Significantly fewer social phobia than panic disorder patients reported palpitations, chest pains, tinnitus, blurred vision, headaches, and fear of dying. Significantly fewer panic disorder than social phobia patients reported dry mouth.

The cognitions of patients with panic disorder with or without agoraphobia center on thoughts of losing bodily control, experiencing a physically catastrophic event, or becoming psychologically disabled. The cognitions of social phobia patients are characterized by fear of negative evaluation and self-depreciation (Turner & Beidel, 1989). Munjack, Brown, and McDowell (1987) found that social phobia patients have greater "interpersonal sensitivity," while panic disorder patients have greater somatization. Amies et al. (1983) also found that social phobia patients score lower on "extraversion" than agoraphobia patients.

Gelernter et al. (1992) found that social phobia patients reported significantly greater levels of social phobic avoidance and distress, fear of negative evaluation, and avoidance of social situations than did panic disorder patients (with and without agoraphobia). The latter reported more overall anxiety and rated themselves as significantly more avoidant of circumstances involving exposure to public places and to blood or injury. The discriminant function analyses showed that social phobia and panic disorder patients can be reliably differentiated on the scales that were used. On all measures assessing social anxiety and avoidance/fear of negative evaluation, the social phobia group consistently scored higher than the panic disorder group. On the scale assessing fear and avoidance of places from which escape might be difficult in the event of panic, the panic disorder group scored significantly higher.

As Uhde et al. (1985, 1991) reported, after an initial uncued panic attack, patients with panic disorder, particularly early in the course of illness, are frightened of subsequent "unpredictable" or "spontaneous" panic attacks, whereas the anxiety of patients with social phobia is cued to social or interpersonal situations.

Some researchers have found a high rate of major depression (63-94%) among patients suffering from panic disorder with comorbid social phobia (Noyes et al., 1992; Reiter, Otto, Pollack, & Rosenbaum, 1991; Stein et al., 1989; Stein, Tancer, & Uhde, 1990). For example, Stein et al. (1989) reported that patients with panic disorder with concomitant social phobia have a remarkably high rate of depression (94%), compared to the rate among patients with panic disorder without social phobia (47%). However, Andersch and Hanson (1993) reported a prevalence for major depression of only 40% in patients with comorbid social phobia and panic disorder, with no significant difference from patients with panic disorder alone. Further studies are needed to resolve this issue.

Help-seeking behavior also clearly distinguishes social phobia patients from panic disorder and agoraphobia patients. Whereas the former often report feeling more comfortable when alone, the latter are comforted by the presence of significant others (Liebowitz, Gorman, et al., 1985). There is even some evidence that panic disorder and agoraphobia patients experience less anxiety when accompanied by familiar figures. In addition, Uhde et al. (1991) reported that during exacerbations of illness, patients with panic disorder seek or demand the support of friends, relatives, or fellow employees, whereas patients with generalized social phobia often retreat into a pattern of social isolation. Furthermore, Schneier, Johnson, et al. (1992) reported that only 5.4% of subjects with uncomplicated social phobia reported seeking services from a mental health practitioner, and only 19.6% reported seeking any outpatient treatment for an emotional problem. In contrast, among ECA study subjects, 72% of those with panic disorder reported seeing a psychiatric professional, and 86% had sought either psychiatric or general medical treatment (Markowitz, Weissman, Ouellete, Lish, & Klerman, 1989). These findings suggest that social phobia is undertreated.

In summary, the best way to distinguish these disorders is based on the nuclear fear and reasons for avoidance. The common thread in social phobia concerns fear of scrutiny, humiliation, and embarrassment. Archetypal examples are speaking, eating, signing one's name in public, and using public lavatories. In panic disorder, however, the primary theme is fear of loss of control, public exposure, or physical or psychological disablement. In agoraphobia, the primary theme is fear of being in places or situations from which escape might be difficult in the event of developing symptoms that could be incapacitating.

Conclusion

It is important to realize, as Brown and Barlow (1992) pointed out, that inclusion of patients in treatment studies on the basis of a given principal diagnosis, without consideration of comorbidity, may give the illusion of sample homogeneity when in fact the sample is quite heterogeneous. Also of importance is the need for systematically evaluating comorbidity.

Regarding the course of illness, it is possible that when social phobia is comorbid with any other disorder, it can promote its characteristic chronic and pervasive style, but future studies are needed to confirm whether this is true. Severity increases in the comorbid situation because of the association itself, the impaired responses to treatment, the reduced help-seeking behavior, and the frequent association with "self-medication" (alcohol and other substance abuse and/or dependence).

In the presence of comorbid disorders, social phobia may be associated with an increased rate of major depression. Comorbid social phobia may also be associated with an increased rate of suicide attempts. Schneier, Johnson, et al. (1992) reported that uncomplicated and comorbid forms of social phobia were associated with increased rates of suicidal ideation. Actual suicide attempts were not associated with uncomplicated social phobia, but in patients with other lifetime psychiatric diagnoses, comorbid social phobia was associated with a nearly six-fold increase in the rate of suicide attempts, compared to persons with no disorder. These findings are consistent with those of other authors (Amies et al., 1983; Davidson et al., 1993; Degonda & Angst, 1993). As Schneier, Johnson, et al. (1992) suggested, persons with social phobia receive inadequate social support, which may be the mechanism by which social phobia interacts with comorbid disorders to increase suicide risk.

Treatment response of the comorbid condition can be informative about the specific linkages and pathophysiology of the co-occurring disorders. If the treatment of the principal diagnosis improves the course of additional diagnoses, the overlap between them is higher than if no influence is seen. Different patterns of response can also be expected in specific comorbid conditions (Carrasco, Hollander, Schneier, & Liebowitz, 1992). This finding suggests a distinctive pathophysiological mechanism of the comorbid situation.

Current evidence suggests that social phobia and panic disorder do not always respond to the same medications or to the same dosages. This may have implications for evaluating the extent to which treatment is effective (Brown & Barlow, 1992), and for establishing what kind of adjustments should be made when comorbidity is present. For example, comorbid generalized social phobia seems to reduce response to serotonin reuptake inhibitors in obsessive-compulsive disorder patients, and MAOIs seem to be an effective alternative medication in such refractory cases (Carrasco et al., 1992). As Carrasco et al. concluded, these findings are consistent with recent reports indicating a decreased rate of response to behavioral treatment among obsessive-compulsive disorder patients who have an associated lack of social skills. Thus deficient social skills as well as distinct biological mechanisms may be involved. We have also noted that while social phobia patients tolerate standard starting dosages of fluoxetine (e.g., 20 mg/day), those with comorbid panic disorder show hypersensitivity and require lower initial dosages (e.g., 5 mg/day).

Social and work impairment increases in the presence of a comorbid condition, but there are still no controlled trials of such conditions. Studies of specific personality traits of comorbid social phobia and panic disorder patients, of the relationship between social anxiety and social phobia, and of the differences between genetic and environmental causes are also necessary. It also is still to be determined whether early treatment of social phobia may affect development of other disorders.

As always with new research fields, the available data on comorbidity are sometimes confusing, for several reasons: There are different clinic samples, community studies, open studies, few controlled studies, different diagnostic systems and scales, and few pathophysiological trials. A common methodological framework is necessary to obtain reliable and comparable data, both in epidemiological and clinical samples. Only then will controlled studies of the impact of comorbidity on phenomenology, diagnosis, course, severity, therapeutics, impairment, and psychopathophysiology be valuable.

Acknowledgment

The authors wish to acknowledge that Tables 1-4 are updated from tables that were originally published in: Mannuzza, S., Fyer, A.J., Liebowitz, M.R., & Klein, D.F. (1990). Delineating the boundaries of social phobia: Its relationship to panic disorder and social phobia. *Journal of Anxiety Disorders, 4,* 41-59.

References

American Psychiatric Association. (1980). *Diagnostic and statistical manual of mental disorders* (3rd ed.). Washington, DC: Author.

American Psychiatric Association. (1987). *Diagnostic and statistical manual of mental disorders* (3rd ed., rev.). Washington, DC: Author.

Amies, P.L., Gelder, M.G., & Shaw, P.M. (1983). Social phobia: A comparative clinical study. *British Journal of Psychiatry, 142,* 174-179.

Andersch, S.E., & Hanson, L.C. (1993). Comorbidity of panic disorder and social phobia. *European Journal of Psychiatry, 7,* 59-64.

Bakish, D. (1994). The use of the reversible monoamine oxidase-A inhibitor brofaromine in social phobia complicated by panic disorder with or without agoraphobia [Letter to the editor]. *Journal of Clinical Psychopharmacology, 14,* 74-75.

Barlow, D.H. (1985). The dimensions of anxiety disorders. In A.H. Tuma & J.D. Maser (Eds.), *Anxiety and the anxiety disorders* (pp. 479-500). Hillsdale, NJ: Erlbaum.

Barlow, D.H., DiNardo, P.A., Vermilyea, B.B., Vermilyea, J., & Blanchard, E.B. (1986). Co-morbidity and depression among the anxiety disorders: Issues in diagnosis and classification. *Journal of Nervous and Mental Disease, 174,* 63-72.

Barlow, D.H., Vermilyea, J., Blanchard, E.B., Vermilyea, B.B., DiNardo, P.A., & Cerny, J.A. (1985). The phenomenon of panic. *Journal of Abnormal Psychology, 94,* 320-328.

Beidel, D.C. (1991). Social phobia and overanxious disorder in school-age children. *Journal of the American Academy of Child and Adolescent Psychiatry, 30,* 545-552.

Black, B., Uhde, T.W., & Tancer, M.E. (1992). Fluoxetine for the treatment of social phobia [Letter to the editor]. *Journal of Clinical Psychopharmacology, 12,* 293-295.

Brown, T.A., & Barlow, D.H. (1992). Comorbidity among anxiety disorders: Implications for treatment and DSM-IV. *Journal of Consulting and Clinical Psychology, 60,* 835-844.

Burke, K.C., Burke, J.D., Regier, D.A., & Rae, D.S. (1990). Age at onset of selected mental disorders in five community populations. *Archives of General Psychiatry, 47,* 511-518.

Burns, L.E., & Thorpe, G.L. (1977). The epidemiology of fears and phobias (with particular reference to the National Survey of Agoraphobics). *Journal of International Medical Research, 5,* 1-7.

Cameron, O.G., Thyer, B.A., Nesse, R.M., & Curtis, G.C. (1986). Symptom profiles of patients with DSM-III anxiety disorders. *American Journal of Psychiatry, 143,* 1132-1137.

Carrasco, J.L., Hollander, E., Schneier, F.R., & Liebowitz, M.R. (1992). Treatment outcome of obsessive compulsive disorder with comorbid social phobia. *Journal of Clinical Psychiatry, 53,* 387-391.

Davidson, J.R.T., Hughes, D.L., George, L.K., & Blazer, D.G. (1993). The epidemiology of social phobia: Findings from the Duke Epidemiological Catchment Area study. *Psychological Medicine, 23,* 709-718.

de Ruiter, C., Rijken, H. Garssen, B., van Schaik, A., & Kraaimaat, F. (1989). Comorbidity among the anxiety disorders. *Journal of Anxiety Disorders, 3,* 57-68.

Degonda, M., & Angst, J. (1993). The Zurich study: XX. Social phobia and agoraphobia. *European Archives of Psychiatry and Clinical Neuroscience, 243,* 95-102.

DiNardo, P.A., & Barlow, D.H. (1990). Syndrome and symptom co-occurrence in the anxiety disorders. In J.D. Maser & C.R. Cloninger (Eds.), *Comorbidity of mood and anxiety disorders* (pp. 205-230). Washington, DC: American Psychiatric Press.

DiNardo, P.A., O'Brien, G.T., Barlow, D.H., Waddell, M.T., & Blanchard, E.B. (1983). Reliability of DSM-III anxiety disorder categories using a new structured interview. *Archives of General Psychiatry, 40,* 1070-1074.

Doctor, R.M. (1982). Major results of a large-scale pretreatment survey of agoraphobics. In R.L. DuPont (Ed.), *Phobia: A comprehensive summary of modern treatments* (pp. 203-214). New York: Brunner/Mazel.

Eaton, W.W., Dryman, A., & Weissman, M.M. (1991). The diagnosis of panic disorder and phobic disorder. In L.N. Robins & D.A. Regier (Eds.), *Psychiatric disorders in America: The Epidemiological Catchment Area study* (pp. 155-179). New York: Free Press.

Feinstein, A.R. (1970). The pre-therapeutic classification of comorbidity in chronic disease. *Journal of Chronic Disease, 23,* 455-468.

Fyer, A.J. (1993). Heritability of social anxiety: A brief review. *Journal of Clinical Psychiatry, 54*(Suppl. 12), 10-12.

Fyer, A.J., Mannuzza, S., Chapman, T.F., Liebowitz, M.R., & Klein, D.F. (1993). A direct interview family study of social phobia. *Archives of General Psychiatry, 50,* 286-293.

Gelernter, C.S., Stein, M.B., Tancer, M.E., & Uhde, T.W. (1992). An examination of syndromal validity and diagnostic subtypes in social phobia and panic disorder. *Journal of Clinical Psychiatry, 53,* 23-27.

Gorman, J.M., Fyer, M.R., Goetz, R., Askanazi, J., Liebowitz, M.R., Fyer, A.J., Kinney, J., & Klein, D.F. (1988). Ventilatory physiology of patients with panic disorder. *Archives of General Psychiatry, 45,* 31-39.

Gorman, J.M.,& Gorman, L.K. (1987). Drug treatment of social phobia. *Journal of Affective Disorders, 13,* 183-192.

Gorman, J.M., Levy, G.F., Liebowitz, M.R., McGrath, P., Appleby, I.L., Dillon, D.J., Davies, S.O., & Klein, D.F. (1983). Effect of acute ß-adrenergic blockage on lactate-induced panic. *Archives of General Psychiatry, 40,* 1079-1082.

Gorman, J.M., Liebowitz, M.R., Fyer, A.J., Goetz, D., Campeas, R.B., Fyer, M.R., Davies, S.O., & Klein, D.F. (1987). An open trial of fluoxetine in the treatment of panic attacks. *Journal of Clinical Psychopharmacology, 7,* 329-332.

Horwath, E., Lish, J.D., Johnson, J., Hornig, C.D., & Weissman, M.M. (1993). Agoraphobia without panic: Clinical reappraisal of an epidemiologic finding. *American Journal of Psychiatry, 150,* 1496-1501.

Kendler, K.S., Neale, M.C., Kessler, R.C., Heath, A.C., & Eaves, L.J. (1992). The genetic epidemiology of phobias in women: The interrelationship of agoraphobia, social phobia, situational phobia, and simple phobia. *Archives of General Psychiatry, 49,* 273-281.

Kessler, R.C., McGonagle, K.A., Zhao, S., Nelson, C.B., Hughes, M., Eshleman, S., Wittchen, H., & Kendler, K.S. (1994). Lifetime and 12-month prevalence of DSM-III-R psychiatric disorders in the United States. *Archives of General Psychiatry, 51,* 8-19.

Klein, D.F. (1964). Delineation of two drug-responsive anxiety syndromes. *Psychopharmacologia, 53,* 397-408.

Klein, D.F. (1991). Anxiety reconceptualized. In D.F. Klein & J. Rabkin (Eds.), *Anxiety: New research and changing concepts* (pp. 235-263). New York: Raven.

Klerman, G.L. (1990). Approaches to the phenomena of comorbidity. In J.D. Maser & C.R. Cloninger (Eds.), *Comorbidity of mood and anxiety disorders* (pp. 13-37). Washington, DC: American Psychiatric Press.

Liebowitz, M.R. (1987). Social phobia. *Modern Problems of Pharmacopsychiatry, 22,* 141-173.

Liebowitz, M.R. (1993). Pharmacotherapy of social phobia. *Journal of Clinical Psychiatry, 54*(12, Suppl.), 31-35.

Liebowitz, M.R., Fyer, A.J., Gorman, J.M., Dillon, D., Davies, S., Stein, J.M., Cohen, B.S., & Klein, D.F. (1985). Specificity of lactate infusions in social phobia versus panic disorders. *American Journal of Psychiatry, 142,* 947-949.

Liebowitz, M.R., Gorman, J.M., Fyer, A.J., & Klein, D.F. (1985). Social phobia: Review of a neglected anxiety disorder. *Archives of General Psychiatry, 42,* 729-736.

Liebowitz, M.R., Schneier, F., Campeas, R., Hollander, E., Hatterer, J., Fyer, A., Gorman, J., Papp, L., Davies, S., Gully, R., & Klein, D.F. (1992). Phenelzine vs atenolol in social phobia: A placebo-controlled comparison. *Archives of General Psychiatry, 49,* 290-300.

Mannuzza, S., Fyer, A.J., Klein, D.F., & Endicott, J. (1986). Schedule for Affective Disorders and Schizophrenia-Lifetime Version modified for the study of anxiety disorders (SADS-LA): Rationale and conceptual development. *Journal of Psychiatric Research, 20,* 317-325.

Mannuzza, S., Fyer, A.J., Liebowitz, M.R., & Klein, D.F. (1990). Delineating the boundaries of social phobia: Its relationship to panic disorder and agoraphobia. *Journal of Anxiety Disorders, 4,* 41-59.

Markowitz, J.S., Weissman, M.M., Ouellette, R., Lish, J.D., & Klerman, G.L. (1989). Quality of life in panic disorder. *Archives of General Psychiatry, 46,* 984-992.

Marks, I.M. (1970). The classification of phobic disorders. *British Journal of Psychiatry, 116,* 377-386.

Marks, I.M., & Gelder, M.G. (1966). Different ages of onset in varieties of phobia. *American Journal of Psychiatry, 123,* 218-221.

Marks, I.M., & Herst, E.R. (1970). A survey of 1,200 agoraphobics in Britain: Features associated with treatment and ability to work. *Social Psychiatry, 5,* 16-24.

Myers., J.K., Weissman, M.M., Tischler, G.L., Holzer, C.E. III, Leaf, P.J., Orvaschel, H., Anthony, J.C., Boyd, J.H., Burke, J.D., Jr., Kramer, M., & Stoltzman, R. (1984). Six-month prevalence of psychiatric disorders in three communities: 1980 to 1982. *Archives of General Psychiatry, 41,* 959-967.

Munjack, D.J., Brown, R.A., & McDowell, D.E. (1987). Comparison of social anxiety in patients with social phobia and panic disorder. *Journal of Nervous and Mental Disease, 175,* 49-51.

Noyes, R., Jr., Anderson, D.J., Clancey, J., Crowe, R.R., Slymen, D.J., Ghoneim, M.M., & Hinrichs, J.V. (1984). Diazepam and propranolol in panic disorder and agoraphobia. *Archives of General Psychiatry, 41,* 287-292.

Noyes, R., Jr., Woodman, C., Garvey, M.J., Cook, B.L., Suelzer, M., Clancy, J., & Anderson, D.J. (1992). Generalized anxiety disorder vs panic disorder: Distinguishing characteristics and patterns of comorbidity. *Journal of Nervous and Mental Disease, 180,* 369-379.

Ost, L.G. (1987). Age of onset in different phobias. *Journal of Abnormal Psychology, 96,* 223-229.

Pollard, C.A., & Cox, G.L. (1988). Social-evaluative anxiety in panic disorder and agoraphobia. *Psychological Reports, 62,* 323-326.

Pollard, C.A., & Henderson, J.G. (1987). Prevalence of agoraphobia: Some confirmatory data. *Psychological Reports, 60,* 1305.

Pollard, C.A.,& Henderson, J.G. (1988). Four types of social phobia in a community sample. *Journal of Nervous and Mental Disease, 176,* 440-445.

Reich, J.H., Noyes, R., & Yates, W. (1988). Anxiety symptoms distinguishing social phobia from panic and generalized anxiety disorders. *Journal of Nervous and Mental Disease, 176,* 510-513.

Reich, J.H., & Yates, W. (1988). Family history of psychiatric disorders in social phobia. *Comprehensive Psychiatry, 29,* 72-75.

Reiter, S.R., Otto, M.W., Pollack, M.H., & Rosenbaum, J.F. (1991). Major depression in panic disorder patients with comorbid social phobia. *Journal of Affective Disorders, 22,* 171-177.

Robins, L.N., Locke, B.Z., & Regier, D.A. (1991). An overview of psychiatric disorders in America. In L.N. Robins & D.A., Regier (Eds.), *Psychiatric disorders in America: The Epidemiologic Catchment Area study* (pp. 328-366). New York: Free Press.

Sanderson, W.C., Rapee, R.M., & Barlow, D.H. (1987, November). *The DSM-III-R revised anxiety disorder categories: Descriptions and patterns of comorbidity.* Paper presented at the annual meeting of the Association for Advancement of Behavior Therapy, Boston.

Sanderson, W.C., DiNardo, P.A., Rapee, R.M., & Barlow, D.H. (1990). Syndrome comorbidity in patients diagnosed with a DSM-III-R anxiety disorder. *Journal of Abnormal Psychology, 99,* 308-312.

Scheibe, G., & Albus, M. (1992). Age at onset, precipitating events, sex distribution, and co-occurrence of anxiety disorders. *Psychopathology, 25,* 11-18.

Schneier, F.R., Chin, S.J., Hollander, E., & Liebowitz, M.R. (1992). Fluoxetine in social phobia [Letter to the editor]. *Journal of Clinical Psychopharmacology, 12,* 62-63.

Schneier, F.R., Johnson, J., Hornig, C.D., Liebowitz, M.R., & Weissman, M.M. (1992). Social phobia: Comorbidity and morbidity in an epidemiologic sample. *Archives of General Psychiatry, 49,* 282-288.

Schneier, F.R., Liebowitz, M.R., Davies, S.O., Fairbanks, J., Hollander, E., Campeas, R., & Klein, D.F. (1990). Fluoxetine in panic disorder. *Journal of Clinical Psychopharmacology, 10,* 119-121.

Shafar, S. (1976). Aspects of phobic illness: A study of 90 personal cases. *British Journal of Medical Psychology, 49,* 221-236.

Sheehan, D.V., Ballenger, J.C., & Jacobsen, G. (1980). Treatment of endogenous anxiety with phobic, hysterical, and hypochondriacal symptoms. *Archives of General Psychiatry, 37,* 51-59.

Sheehan, D.V., Sheehan, K.E., & Minichiello, W.E. (1981). Age of onset of phobic disorders: A reevaluation. *Comprehensive Psychiatry, 22,* 544-553.

Solyom, L., Ledwidge, B., & Solyom, C. (1986). Delineating social phobia. *British Journal of Psychiatry, 149,* 464-470.

Starcevic, V., Uhlenhuth, E.H., Kellner, R., & Pathak. (1992). Patterns of comorbidity in panic disorder and agoraphobia. *Psychiatry Research, 42,* 171-183.

Stein, M.B., Shea, C.A., & Uhde, T.W. (1989). Social phobic symptoms in patients with panic disorder: Practical and theoretical implications. *American Journal of Psychiatry, 146,* 235-238.

Stein, M.B., Tancer, M.E., & Uhde, T.W. (1990). Major depression in patients with panic disorder: Factors associated with course and recurrence. *Journal of Affective Disorders, 19,* 287-296.

Tancer, M.E. (1993). Neurobiology of social phobia. *Journal of Clinical Psychiatry, 54*(12, Suppl.), 26-30.

Telch, M.J., Brouillard, M., Telch, C.F., Agras, W.S., & Taylor, C.B. (1989). Role of cognitive appraisal in panic-related avoidance. *Behaviour Research and Therapy, 27,* 373-383.

Tesar, G.E., Rosenbaum, J.F., Pollack, M.H., Otto, M.W., Sachs, G.S., Herman, J.B., Cohen, L.S., & Spier, S.A. (1991). Double-blind, placebo-controlled comparison of clonazepam and alprazolam for panic disorder. *Journal of Clinical Psychiatry, 52,* 69-76.

Thyer, B.A., Parrish, R.T., Curtis, G.C., Nesse, R.M., & Cameron, O.G. (1985). Ages of onset of DSM-III anxiety disorders. *Comprehensive Psychiatry, 26,* 113-122.

Turner, S.M., & Beidel, D.C. (1989). Social phobia: Clinical syndrome, diagnosis, and comorbidity. *Clinical Psychology Review, 9,* 3-18.

Turner, S.M., Beidel, D.C., Dancu, C.V., & Keys, D.J. (1986). Psychopathology of social phobia and comparison to avoidant personality disorder. *Journal of Abnormal Psychology, 95,* 389-394.

Uhde, T.W., Tancer, M.E., Black, B., & Brown, T.M. (1991). Phenomenology and neurobiology of social phobia: Comparison with panic disorder. *Journal of Clinical Psychiatry, 52*(11, Suppl.), 31-40.

Van Ameringen, M., Mancini, C., & Streiner, D.L. (1993). Fluoxetine efficacy in social phobia. *Journal of Clinical Psychiatry, 54,* 27-32.

Van Ameringen, M., Mancini, C., Styan, G., & Donison, D. (1991). Relationship of social phobia with other psychiatric illness. *Journal of Affective Disorders, 21,* 93-99.

Wittchen, H.U., Essau, C.A., & Krieg, J.C. (1991). Anxiety disorders: Similarities and differences of comorbidity in treated and untreated groups. *British Journal of Psychiatry, 159*(Suppl. 12), 23-33.

3. Comorbidity in Social Phobia: Implications for Cognitive-Behavioral Treatment

David H. Barlow, PhD

On the basis of several decades of research at our center and elsewhere on the nature of anxiety, we have developed a model of anxiety suggesting that this mood state is best described as a loose, cognitive, affective structure. In this model, anxiety is composed primarily of high negative affect associated with a sense of the uncontrollability of future events. The sense that events in one's life are out of control is focused primarily on future threat, danger, or the possible occurrence of other negative events. This negative affect is also associated with a shift in attention to a self-evaluative mode, or a state of self-preoccupation.

This negative affective state can also be described as "helplessness," because individuals suffering from severe anxiety consistently perceive an inability on their part to predict, control, or obtain desired results in upcoming situations and turn their attention inward to monitor their (inadequate) response state. Almost anyone describing personal anxiety would say something like, "That terrible event is not my fault, but it may happen (again), and even though I probably can't cope with it, I've got to be ready to try" (Barlow, 1988, 1991). Because this state of negative affect is oriented toward future events rather than present reality, the term we have come to use is "anxious apprehension"—a term we consider synonymous with anxiety. The state of readiness or preparation for future negative events that characterizes anxious apprehension is best reflected in the chronic tension and arousal that seem so characteristic of anxiety (Marten et al., 1993). Such arousal and central nervous system tension may well be the physiological substrate of "readiness" that underlies any effort to counteract potentially uncontrollable upcoming events (Fridlund, Hatfield, Cottam, & Fowler, 1986). Accompanying this sense of uncontrollability and associated physical state of readiness is a vigilance (or hypervigilance) for cues or signals that may presage upcoming negative events. The process of anxiety based on this model is presented in Figure 1.

With specific reference to this figure, a variety of cues or "propositions" (in the words of the emotion theorist Peter Lang, 1985) would be sufficient to evoke anxious apprehension. Furthermore, such anxi-

---

Dr. Barlow is distinguished professor of psychology at the University at Albany, State University of New York, Albany.

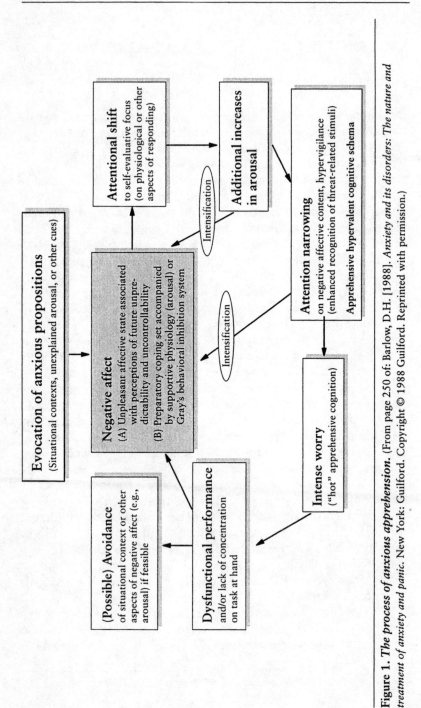

Figure 1. *The process of anxious apprehension.* (From page 250 of: Barlow, D.H. [1988]. *Anxiety and its disorders: The nature and treatment of anxiety and panic.* New York: Guilford. Copyright © 1988 Guilford. Reprinted with permission.)

ety would be, in many cases, "unconscious" because it occurs without the need for conscious, rational appraisal. The cues may be very broad, as in the case of social evaluation anxiety, or very narrow, as would be the case with test anxiety or sexual dysfunction. In the latter case, anxious apprehension would occur only if a formal test or a sexual union was imminent.

The attentional shift to a self-evaluative focus is often referred to clinically as neurotic self-preoccupation. In fact, focus of attention seems to shift very rapidly from external sources of potential threat to an internal self-evaluative mode (Barlow, 1988). Some aspects of the body of knowledge regarding self-focused attention are relevant not only to anxiety, but also to the development of social anxiety and social phobia. First, we know that self-focused attention increases sensitivity to bodily sensations and other sources of internal experience. This sensitivity to bodily sensations seems to spread rapidly to other aspects of the self such as self-evaluative concerns (Carver & Scheier, 1981; Scheier, Carver, & Matthews, 1983). We also know that this tendency to focus internally results directly in a greater subjective intensity of emotional experience. An additional consequence of self-focused attention is a failure to habituate to external stimuli. As one can see in Figure 1, self-focused attention is depicted as generating its own small positive feedback loop, which contributes to an escalation of negative affect and the associated physical concomitants of anxious apprehension. Additional evidence suggests that self-focused attention may be particularly virulent in terms of exacerbating anxious apprehension if the focus is on the affective qualities of the experience, particularly if the affect is negative (Scheier et al., 1983).

In any case, the arousal associated with the process of anxious apprehension may lead to a dramatic narrowing of attention on the focus of threat or anxiety and may also contribute to the sense that one may not be able to cope with the upcoming threat. Because the arousal (and tension) inherent in this process is not in and of itself problematic (the same arousal also seems to be present in more positive emotions such as excitement), it is the sense of uncontrollability and the tendency to focus internally along with narrowed attention that seem more related to the types of deficits that appear in social phobia and other anxiety disorders. In its extreme state, this process may lead to a runaway positive feedback loop characterized by intense "worry" that individuals are unable to shut off or control in any effective way. This arousal-driven worry may in turn lead to disruptions in concentration—one of the hallmarks of clinical anxiety. In social situations, this process may lead to disruptions in performance.

When applied to social anxiety and social phobia, the cues or propositions evoking anxious apprehension are, of course, social. These cues might include demands for social performance or interaction, which leads to the elicitation of negative affect and expectancies, an internal focus on the consequences of performing poorly in social situations, increased arousal, a narrowing of attention, and, ultimately, deteriorated performance in these social situations (see Figure 2).

It is important to recognize that one of the potentially dangerous and uncontrollable events occurring in a social situation could be a situationally bound panic attack. That is, as specified in *DSM-IV*, an initial unexpected panic attack in a social situation may become highly likely to recur in subsequent social situations through a process of conditioning and generalization. Thus the panic attack would not be "unexpected" in that it would not occur outside these social situations but would instead be situationally bound or at least situationally predisposed. In the latter case, the patient might not always be able to predict when the panic attack would occur in a specific social situation, only that it would be likely to occur at some point. Thus anxious apprehension becomes focused not only on the possible threat of embarrassing oneself due to poor performance or related concerns, but also on the possibility of experiencing an uncontrollable panic attack in this situation (Barlow, 1988, 1992). In any case, it is this model of anxiety and social phobia that has driven the development of cognitive-behavioral treatment in our setting (e.g., Hope & Heimberg, 1993).

The Albany Social Phobia Program

The program developed at our center in Albany is administered in a group setting, most often by two cotherapists. Typically, five social phobia patients participate in the treatment protocol, which is administered weekly for approximately 3 months. The treatment has five components. The first three components are: (1) education about social phobia from a cognitive-behavioral perspective, (2) the elicitation and analysis of specific cognitions that are relevant to danger and threat in socially phobic situations, and (3) exposure to anxiety-provoking situations in the context of group therapy. These anxiety-provoking situations are usually simulated real-life encounters using other members in the group as well as the cotherapists in a role-playing format. The final two components are: (4) cognitive restructuring procedures that target relevant negative cognitions concerning the social situation both before, during, and after the simulated exposure exercises, and (5) homework assignments in which the patient uses

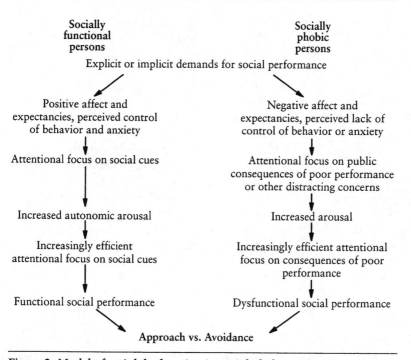

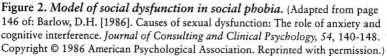

Figure 2. *Model of social dysfunction in social phobia.* (Adapted from page 146 of: Barlow, D.H. [1986]. Causes of sexual dysfunction: The role of anxiety and cognitive interference. *Journal of Consulting and Clinical Psychology, 54,* 140-148. Copyright © 1986 American Psychological Association. Reprinted with permission.)

newly developed cognitive and behavioral procedures to cope with anxiety and naturally occurring socially phobic situations (Barlow, 1992; Hope & Heimberg, 1993). Specific components of this structured approach to therapy are scheduled in Session 1, Session 2, and Sessions 3-11 (see Tables 1, 2, and 3).

This program has been evaluated in a number of studies at our center, some of which are still ongoing. In the first of several studies, Heimberg, Becker, Goldfinger, and Vermilyea (1985) treated seven relatively severe social phobia patients. At the end of the 14-week treatment, all subjects had improved substantially. At 6-month follow-up, six of the seven subjects had maintained their improvement. Later studies used a "psychological placebo" meant to control for the nonspecific effects of the Albany Social Phobia protocol. The psychological placebo, referred to as educational supportive group therapy (ES), consists of education on the nature of social phobia, extensive discussion of socially phobic situations, and nonspecific support in the context of group therapy. Participating patients rate this protocol as highly credible both before and after treatment. In the first comparison of the Albany Social Phobia protocol with ES (Heimberg et al., 1990), patients in both treatments were significantly improved on most measures immediately following treatment. Patients receiving the Albany Social Phobia protocol, however, showed greater improvement on key measures of social phobia, including reports of anxiety during individualized behavior assessments, and on clinical ratings of social phobia severity by an independent evaluator. More importantly, patients who received the social phobia protocol were more likely to maintain their gains and showed significantly more improvement than individuals in the ES condition at a 5-year follow-up (Heimberg, Salzman, Holt, & Blendell, 1993).

A multicenter study is now being conducted to compare the Albany protocol to an effective drug treatment (phenelzine), along with pill placebo and the ES condition. All four treatment conditions are ongoing at two different sites, the Center for Stress and Anxiety Disorders in Albany and the New York State Psychiatric Institute (Heimberg & Liebowitz, 1992). Blinded, independent assessors have now rated the first 77 individuals who have completed treatment, categorizing them either as responders or nonresponders. According to preliminary data, patients receiving either active psychosocial treatment or phenelzine have done comparably well; 80% of the subjects receiving the Albany Social Phobia protocol were rated as responders, as were 71% of those receiving phenelzine. Improvement

Table 1. *Outline of Cognitive-Behavioral Group Therapy procedures for Session 1*

1. Complete Beck Depression Inventory and any other optional questionnaire(s).
2. Make introductions.
3. Review basic ground rules [therapists].
4. Share social fears and goals for treatment [each member].
5. Describe cognitive-behavioral model for social phobia and rationale for treatment [therapists].
6. Provide initial training in cognitive restructuring.
   a. Exercise 1: Therapist relates personal situation.
   b. Exercise 2: Group members share automatic thoughts regarding coming to group for the first time.
7. Assign homework.

(Reprinted from page 113 of: Hope, D., & Heimberg, R.G. [1993]. Social phobia and social anxiety. In D.H. Barlow [Ed.], *Clinical handbook of psychological disorders* [2nd ed., pp. 99–136]. New York: Guilford. Copyright © 1993 Guilford. Reprinted with permission.)

Table 2. *Outline of Cognitive-Behavioral Group Therapy procedures for Session 2*

1. Complete Beck Depression Inventory and any other optional questionnaire(s).
2. Review homework from previous week.
3. Continue training in cognitive restructuring.
   a. Therapists introduce concept of "cognitive distortion."
   b. Exercise 3: Group identifies distortion in automatic thoughts from homework.
   c. Therapists introduce dispute handles and rational responses.
   d. Exercise 4: Imaginal scenario.
   e. Exercise 5: Group challenges automatic thoughts from homework and develops rational responses.
4. Assign homework.

(Reprinted from page 114 of: Hope, D., & Heimberg, R.G. [1993]. Social phobia and social anxiety. In D.H. Barlow [Ed.], *Clinical handbook of psychological disorders* [2nd ed., pp. 99-136]. New York: Guilford. Copyright © 1993 Guilford. Reprinted with permission.)

Table 3. *Outline of Cognitive-Behavioral Group Therapy procedures for Sessions 3-11*

1. Complete Beck Depression Inventory and any other optional questionnaire(s).
2. Review homework from previous week.
3. Complete three in-session exposures.
   a. Select target group member and briefly outline exposure situation.
   b. Elicit automatic thoughts.
   c. Pick one or two thoughts to pursue further.
   d. Label cognitive distortion(s) in selected automatic thought(s).
   e. Challenge selected automatic thought(s) using the dispute handles.
   f. Develop one or two rational responses.
   g. Develop details of the exposure situations.
   h. Set a nonperfectionistic, behavioral goal.
   i. Complete role play.
   j. Debrief exposure.
      1. Review goal attainment.
      2. Carry out other activities as appropriate.
4. Assign homework.

(Reprinted from page 114 of: Hope, D., & Heimberg, R.G. [1993]. Social phobia and social anxiety. In D.H. Barlow [Ed.], *Clinical handbook of psychological disorders* [2nd ed., pp. 99-136]. New York: Guilford. Copyright © 1993 Guilford. Reprinted with permission.)

rates in both groups were significantly higher than for those patients receiving pill placebo (37%) or psychosocial placebo (ES, 27%). These data indicate that effective treatments, both drug and psychosocial, are available for individuals suffering from severe social phobia. Recent updated analyses do not change the pattern of results.

Comorbidity and social phobia

Despite these encouraging results, analyses of the perplexing problem of comorbidity and its effects on treatment have only begun. One can study comorbidity either cross-sectionally or longitudinally. When studying comorbidity in a cross-sectional analysis, one simply takes a snapshot of diagnostic conditions co-occurring at a specific point in time (during the interview). A longitudinal analysis, which may in the long run be more theoretically fruitful, entails examining the full range of disorders an individual has experienced during a lifetime and the chronological relationship of these disorders. Rates of cross-sectional comorbidity derived from a large sample of 468 consecutively diagnosed patients who presented for evaluation at our center revealed extensive comorbidity. In this sample, both principal and additional diagnoses were made after administering the Anxiety Disorders Interview Schedule–Revised (ADIS-R, DiNardo & Barlow, 1988), an instrument capable of yielding reliable diagnoses among anxiety and related disorders in the hands of trained interviewers. For example, kappa coefficients for social phobia are .79 when social phobia is the principal diagnosis, and .66 when social phobia is either the principal or an additional diagnosis (DiNardo, Moras, Barlow, Rapee, & Brown, 1993). Principal diagnosis in this case refers to the diagnosis judged by the interviewer to be associated with the greatest degree of distress or impairment. In fact, 50% of patients with a principal anxiety disorder had at least one clinically significant comorbid anxiety or depressive disorder. These findings generally are consistent with previous studies (e.g., de Ruiter, Rijken, Garssen, van Schaik, & Kraaimaat, 1989; Sanderson, DiNardo, Rapee, & Barlow, 1990). Across all patients, generalized anxiety disorder (GAD) was the most frequently assigned additional diagnosis at a clinically significant level (23%); it was followed by social phobia (14%). Interestingly, GAD and social phobia were also the most frequently assigned additional diagnoses in another study consisting of patients identified with a principal mood disorder (Sanderson, Beck, & Beck, 1990).

When social phobia is the principal (or most severe) disorder, it may be comorbid with a range of other anxiety or mood disorders. According to data from a study of 76 patients consecutively diagnosed as having social phobia (see Table 4), all of whom received the ADIS-R, fully 17% of the social phobia patients had an additional diagnosis of generalized anxiety disorder and 20% presented with an additional mood

48

Table 4. *Percentages of additional diagnoses among patients with social phobia*

Additional diagnoses	Social phobia (N = 76)
Anxiety disorders	
Panic disorder	4
Panic disorder with mild agoraphobia	4
Panic disorder with moderate agoraphobia	1
Panic disorder with severe agoraphobia	0
Social phobia	
Generalized anxiety disorder	17
Obsessive-compulsive disorder	1
Simple phobia	9
Mood disorders	
Major depressive episode	11
Dysthymia	13
Major depressive episode or dysthymia	20

(Adapted from page 838 of: Brown, T.A., & Barlow, D.H. [1992]. Comorbidity among anxiety disorders: Implications for treatment and DSM-IV. *Journal of Consulting and Clinical Psychology, 60,* 835-844. Copyright © 1992 American Psychological Association. Reprinted with permission.)

disorder, either a major depressive episode or dysthymia (Brown & Barlow, 1992). Once again, these comorbidity rates are based on additional diagnoses of clinically significant proportions. In other words, these diagnoses all met the threshold for "caseness." Diagnoses not meeting this threshold of impairment (referred to as subclinical diagnoses) were not included, but previous studies indicate that rates of comorbidity would increase substantially if subclinical diagnoses were included in the calculations (Sanderson, DiNardo, et al., 1990). In fact, if social fears and phobias are considered symptoms rather than a disorder, then these symptoms are widely distributed among the anxiety disorders (Rapee, Sanderson, & Barlow, 1988), as are symptoms of panic (Barlow et al., 1985). These data suggest that another possible way of organizing this information would be to rate symptoms of panic or social anxiety dimensionally to ascertain relative severity of these features in any patient presenting with an anxiety disorder and, possibly, a mood disorder (Barlow, 1988; Moras & Barlow, 1992).

Yet another set of interesting data on comorbidity comes from a recent study by Schwalberg and Barlow (1992), which examined the incidence of comorbid anxiety disorders among a group of eating disorder patients. The investigators noted that a striking proportion of eating disorder patients were comorbid for one or more anxiety disorders. The most frequent comorbid disorders were, once again, generalized anxiety disorder and social phobia. Fully 40% of a group of patients presenting with bulimia nervosa evidenced social phobia, as did 36.4% of another group of obese binge eaters.

Implications of comorbidity for treatment

Data are beginning to accumulate on the effects of existing comorbidity on treatment outcome, either psychosocial or pharmacological. Although we have not yet examined the effect of comorbid conditions on outcome during the treatment of social phobia, we have looked at the effects of a comorbid social phobia diagnosis on outcome during treatment of panic disorder (see Figure 3). Specifically, the presence of an additional diagnosis of social phobia did not have a substantial impact on the outcome of treatment for panic disorder. In fact, in a somewhat anomalous finding, patients with panic disorder and an additional diagnosis of social phobia improved somewhat more than patients with panic disorder without an additional diagnosis of social phobia. However, these differences had disappeared at a 3-month follow-up, at which time both groups were equally improved. More interestingly, from another perspective, we have recently examined the fate of panic disorder patients with a comorbid diagnosis of generalized anxiety disorder who were treated with a successful psychosocial treatment developed specifically for panic disorder, "panic control treatment" (PCT) (Barlow, 1992). In fact, approximately 80% of the individuals in this sample were panic free after treatment (see Figure 4), which is similar to previous results in treating panic disorder with this approach (Barlow, Craske, Cerny, & Klosko, 1989). As Figure 4 shows, 32.4% of the patients with a principal diagnosis of panic disorder presented with an additional diagnosis of GAD at a level of clinical severity, while 8.8% presented with subclinical GAD, and 58.8% presented with no evidence of GAD. At posttreatment, the percentage of patients with a diagnosis of GAD dropped to 8.8%; this relatively low percentage was maintained at 3-month follow-up. Thus treatment for panic disorder seemed to generalize positively to an additional diagnosis of GAD. At present, we are collecting similar data on the fate of social phobia as an additional diagnosis.

Implications

A firm database now exists to suggest that personality disorders, substance abuse, and additional anxiety and mood disorders often ac-

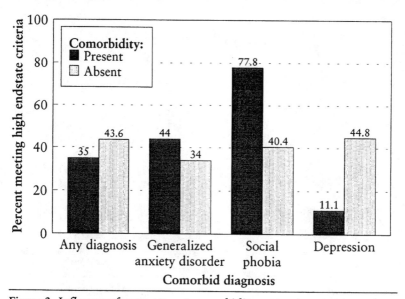

Figure 3. *Influence of pretreatment comorbidity on treatment outcome (posttreatment).* (From: Brown, T.A., Antony, M., Cote, G., & Barlow, D.H. [November, 1992]. *Cognitive-behavioral treatment of panic disorder: Impact and course of comorbid diagnoses.* Paper presented at the annual meeting of the Association for Advancement of Behavior Therapy, Boston, MA.)

company social phobia. Unfortunately, data do not now exist on the possible impact of these comorbid conditions on treatment outcome of social phobia, either with drugs or with psychosocial treatment. Treatment decisions at this time are therefore based primarily on clinical judgment. Data that do exist regarding other disorders suggest that additional anxiety and mood disorders may not pose a particular problem for treatment of target anxiety disorders such as social phobia—because the most common pattern is that these existing comorbid disorders also benefit from treatment, or at least do not detract from the effects of treatment (Brown & Barlow, 1992; Foa, Steketee, Kozak, & McCarthy, 1992).

On the other hand, at least one study (Turner, 1987) suggests that co-occurring personality disorders may predict poor response to behavioral treatment of social phobia. Other studies (Mavissakalian & Hamann, 1986; Noyes et al., 1990) also indicate that personality disorders may predict a poor response of panic disorder to behavioral treatment. There is a clear need to collect more data on the effects of comorbid conditions on treatment of social phobia so that clinical decisions may be data driven rather than based on clinical judgment.

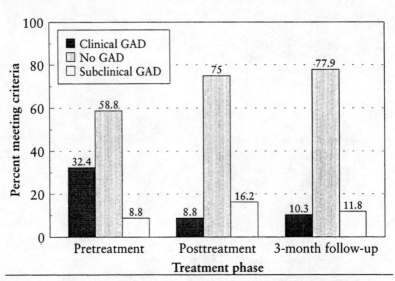

Figure 4. *Effects of panic control treatment on comorbid generalized anxiety disorder (GAD) diagnosis in 68 patients with panic disorder.* (From page 842 of: Brown, T.A., & Barlow, D.H. [1992]. Comorbidity among anxiety disorders: Implications for treatment and DSM-IV. *Journal of Consulting and Clinical Psychology, 60,* 835-844. Copyright © 1992 American Psychological Association. Reprinted with permission.)

Particularly important will be further studies ascertaining how treatment should be adjusted in the presence of comorbid conditions. Results of these studies will also reflect generally on the nature of anxiety and anxiety disorders because the extent to which specific treatments, either psychosocial or drug, have either broadband or narrow effects on the variety of symptomatology presenting in highly comorbid patients will shed light on the relation of the various cognitive, behavioral, and somatic symptoms of anxiety. Comorbidity may also have implications for evaluating the effects of treatment. For example, broad-based improvement in functioning, a common outcome variable, may not be apparent in highly comorbid patients even if the target condition evidences substantial improvement. In other words, alleviation of social phobia may not necessarily generalize to comorbid depression, thus leaving overall functioning in a relatively deteriorated state. In this case, the effects of treatment on social phobia might be underestimated.

For clinical purposes, the best strategy at the current time is to treat social phobia directly if it presents as the principal diagnosis and to carefully observe the effects on comorbid conditions. Based on preliminary data from our studies with panic disorder patients, the most likely possibility is that the comorbid condition will also evidence some improvement. Residual symptoms could then be attacked directly. If, on the other hand, there is no lessening of social phobia, the clinician would certainly want to examine patterns of comorbidity more closely to ascertain whether a comorbid condition might be interfering with what we know to be effective treatment. Patterns of substance abuse and severe personality disorders likely to result in noncompliance with treatment are obvious candidates.

References

Barlow, D.H. (1988). *Anxiety and its disorders: The nature and treatment of anxiety and panic*. NY: Guilford.

Barlow, D.H. (1991). The nature of anxiety: Anxiety, depression, and emotional disorders. In R.M. Rapee & D.H. Barlow (Eds.), *Chronic anxiety: Generalized anxiety disorder and mixed anxiety-depression* (pp. 1-28). New York: Guilford.

Barlow, D.H. (1992). Cognitive-behavioral approaches to panic disorder and social phobia. *Bulletin of the Menninger Clinic, 56*(2, Suppl. A), A14-A28.

Barlow, D.H., Craske, M.G., Cerny, J.A., & Klosko, J.S. (1989). Behavioral treatment of panic disorder. *Behavior Therapy, 20*, 261-282.

Barlow, D.H., Vermilyea, J., Blanchard, E.B., Vermilyea, B.B., DiNardo, P.A., & Cerny, J.A. (1985). The phenomenon of panic. *Journal of Abnormal Psychology, 94*, 320-328.

Brown, T.A., & Barlow, D.H. (1992). Comorbidity among anxiety disorders: Implications for treatment and DSM-IV. *Journal of Consulting and Clinical Psychology, 60*, 835-844.

Carver, C.S., & Scheier, M.F. (1981). *Attention and self-regulation: A control-theory approach to human behavior*. New York: Springer-Verlag.

de Ruiter, C., Rijken, H., Garssen, B., van Schaik, A., & Kraaimaat, F. (1989). Comorbidity among the anxiety disorders. *Journal of Anxiety Disorders, 3*, 57-68.

DiNardo, P.A., & Barlow, D.H. (1988). *Anxiety Disorders Interview Schedule–Revised (ADIS-R)*. Albany, NY: Graywind.

DiNardo, P.A., Moras, K., Barlow, D.H., Rapee, R.M., & Brown, T.A. (1993). Reliability of the DSM-III-R anxiety disorder categories: Using the Anxiety Disorders Interview Schedule–Revised. *Archives of General Psychiatry, 50*, 251-256.

Foa, E., Steketee, G.S., Kozak, M.J., & McCarthy, P.R. (1992). Treatment of depressive and obsessive-compulsive symptoms in OCD by imipramine and behaviour therapy. *British Journal of Clinical Psychology, 31*, 279-292.

Fridlund, A.J., Hatfield, M.E., Cottam, G.L., & Fowler, S.C. (1986). Anxiety and striate-muscle activation: Evidence from electromyographic pattern analysis. *Journal of Abnormal Psychology, 95*, 228-236.

Heimberg, R.G., Becker, R.E., Goldfinger, K., & Vermilyea, J.A. (1985). Treatment of social phobia by exposure, cognitive restructuring, and homework assignments. *Journal of Nervous and Mental Disease, 173*, 236-245.

Heimberg, R.G., Dodge, C.S., Hope, D.A., Kennedy, C.R., Zollo, L., & Becker, R.E. (1990). Cognitive-behavioral group treatment for social phobia: Comparison with a credible placebo control. *Cognitive Therapy and Research, 14*, 1-23.

Heimberg, R.G., & Liebowitz, M.R. (1992, April). *A multi-center comparison of the efficacy of phenelzine and cognitive-behavioral group treatment for social phobia.* Paper presented at the 12th National Conference on Anxiety Disorders, Houston.

Heimberg, R.G., Salzman, D.G., Holt, C.S., & Blendell, K.A. (1993). Cognitive-behavioral group treatment for social phobia: Effectiveness at five-year followup. *Cognitive Therapy and Research, 17,* 325-339.

Hope, D., & Heimberg, R.G. (1993). Social phobia and social anxiety. In D.H. Barlow (Ed.), *Clinical handbook of psychological disorders* (2nd ed., pp. 99-136). New York: Guilford.

Lang, P.J. (1985). The cognitive psychophysiology of emotion: Fear and anxiety. In A.H. Tuma & J.D. Maser (Eds.), *Anxiety and the anxiety disorders* (pp. 131-170). Hillsdale, NJ: Erlbaum.

Marten, P.A., Brown, T.A., Barlow, D.H., Borkovec, T.D., Shear, M.K., & Lydiard, R.B. (1993). Evaluation of the ratings comprising the associated symptom criterion of DSM-III-R generalized anxiety disorder. *Journal of Nervous and Mental Disease, 181,* 676-682.

Mavissakalian, M., & Hamann, M.S. (1986). Assessment and significance of behavioral avoidance in agoraphobia. *Journal of Psychopathology and Behavioral Assessment, 8,* 317-327.

Moras, K., & Barlow, D.H. (1992). Dimensional approaches to diagnosis and the problem of anxiety and depression. In W. Fiegenbaum, A. Ehlers, J. Margraf, & I. Florin (Eds.), *Perspectives and promises of clinical psychology* (pp. 23-37). New York: Plenum.

Noyes, R., Reich, J., Christiansen, J., Suelzer, M., Pfohl, B., & Coryell, W.A. (1990). Outcome of panic disorder: Relationship to diagnostic subtypes and comorbidity. *Archives of General Psychiatry, 47,* 809-818.

Rapee, R.M., Sanderson, W.C., & Barlow, D. H. (1988). Social phobia features across the DSM-III-R anxiety disorders. *Journal of Psychopathology and Behavioral Assessment, 10,* 287-299.

Sanderson, W.C., Beck, A.T., & Beck, J. (1990). Syndrome comorbidity in patients with major depression or dysthymia: Prevalence and temporal relationships. *American Journal of Psychiatry, 147,* 1025-1028.

Sanderson, W.C., DiNardo, P.A., Rapee, R.M., & Barlow, D.H. (1990). Syndrome comorbidity in patients diagnosed with a DSM-III-R anxiety disorder. *Journal of Abnormal Psychology, 99,* 308-312.

Scheier, M.F., Carver, C.S., & Matthews, K.A. (1983). Attentional factors in the perception of bodily states. In J.T. Cacioppo & R.E. Petty (Eds.), *Social psychophysiology: A sourcebook* (pp. 510-542). New York: Guilford.

Schwalberg, M., & Barlow, D.H. (1992). Comparison of bulimics, obese binge eaters, social phobics, and individuals with panic disorder on comorbidity across DSM-III-R anxiety disorders. *Journal of Abnormal Psychology, 101,* 675-681.

Turner, R.M. (1987). The effects of personality disorder diagnosis on the outcome of social anxiety symptom reduction. *Journal of Personality Disorders, 1,* 136-143.

4. The Diagnosis and Treatment of Social Phobia and Alcohol Abuse

John R. Marshall, MD

While the lifetime prevalence of alcohol abuse and dependence in the general population has recently been estimated at 13.5-14.1%, clinical experience bolstered by studies from a variety of settings indicates that there are even higher rates of alcohol-related problems among patients with anxiety disorders (Kessler et al., 1994; Regier et al., 1990; Ross, Glaser, & Germanson, 1988). Some of these studies evaluated anxiety disorders in alcohol treatment settings. In an excellent review and discussion article, Kushner, Sher, and Beitman (1990) summarized studies of alcoholic inpatients and found that estimates of those with anxiety disorders ranged from 22.6% to 68.7%. In another study, Ross et al. (1988) found that 33% of a mixed population of alcoholic inpatients and outpatients currently met criteria for an anxiety disorder. Data from the Epidemiologic Catchment Area (ECA) community survey indicated that 19.4% of patients with alcohol problems suffered an anxiety condition (Regier et al., 1990).

A second group of studies has been done in psychiatric treatment settings. Using *DSM-II* criteria (anxiety neuroses), two studies revealed comorbid rates of 16% and 25%, respectively, of alcohol-related problems (Winokur & Holemon, 1963; Woodruff, Guze, & Clayton, 1972). Using the Michigan Alcoholic Screening Test (MAST) on 156 outpatients diagnosed with *DSM-III* anxiety disorders, Thyer et al. (1986) found that 17.3% scored in the alcoholic range. Studies from the general population reassure us that these comorbidity figures are not simply due to an artifact of sample self-selection (i.e., treatment seeking). The ECA community data pointed to a lifetime prevalence of 17.1% of any alcohol diagnosis among patients with anxiety disorders (Regier et al., 1990). The authors commented that this overall rate is heavily weighted by the high prevalence of phobias, particularly simple phobias, which obscures much higher rates for the less common anxiety conditions.

Social phobia and alcoholism

The types of studies that delineate or specifically focus on social phobia and alcohol problems arise from similar settings. Mullaney and Trippett (1979) found 56% of their alcoholic inpatients to be "fully

---

Dr. Marshall is director of the Anxiety Disorders Center, University of Wisconsin Hospital and Clinics, Madison.

or borderline" socially phobic. Smail, Stockwell, Canter, and Hodgson (1984) determined that 39% of their patients were socially phobic during their last drinking period. Among 75 alcoholic inpatients, Chambless, Cherney, Caputo, and Rheinstein (1987) found that 21% had a history of social phobia. In Ross et al.'s (1988) study of patients with alcohol and other drug-related problems, 12% of the patients met criteria for social phobia. Conversely, Schneier, Martin, Liebowitz, Gorman, and Fyer (1989) examined 98 subjects meeting *DSM-III-R* criteria for social phobia and found that 16.3% (20% of the men, 13% of the women) met Research Diagnostic Criteria for a lifetime diagnosis of alcoholism. This finding probably underestimated the prevalence of alcoholism in the general population of socially phobic individuals because patients who were currently abusing alcohol were excluded from the study.

The comorbid relationship

It seems to be an inescapable conclusion that there is a high rate of comorbidity between social phobia and excessive alcohol intake. In almost all studies of anxiety disorders, social phobia ranks first or second in this association (agoraphobia is also highly correlated). Kushner et al. (1990) summarized the problem by noting that patients with social phobia are more than twice as likely to have alcohol problems as are individuals in the community. They also noted that social phobia is nine times more likely to be present among persons with alcohol disorders than would be expected in the general community.

In our anxiety clinic, social phobia patients who use alcohol moderately to excessively clearly describe the deliberate use of alcohol to reduce social anxiety (i.e., self-medication). Other investigators have noted similar patient descriptions (Bibb & Chambless, 1986; Chambless et al., 1987; Schneier et al., 1989; Smail et al., 1984). It has been observed in multiple studies, consistent with a self-medication explanation, that the social phobia occurred prior to alcohol abuse and/or dependence. This pattern of onset prior to excessive alcohol use is especially true for social phobia and agoraphobia, less often for simple phobias, and distinctly less often for panic disorder and generalized anxiety. For these latter disorders, many patients report the onset of anxiety symptoms concurrent with problematic drinking or after it has been present for a prolonged period. Although it is common for patients with panic disorder and/or agoraphobia to report a worsening of symptoms after drinking, in our experience more severe symptoms are relatively rare among social phobia patients. Of course, after years of the coexistence of both disorders, accurate self-reporting of symptom sequences becomes blurred.

Why social phobia and alcohol?

Despite our long-standing awareness of the anxiolytic properties of alcohol, we do not fully understand the association of these disorders. Early, general theories of alcoholism suggested that the reinforcing properties of alcohol occur by reducing avoidance in approach-avoidance conflict situations (Conger, 1956). Variations of "tension reduction" hypotheses have also been offered (Cappell & Herman, 1972). Others described "stress-response dampening" to threatening stimuli (Sher, 1988). These theories appear plausible, but lack specificity. They neither pinpoint specific adverse emotional states (i.e., fear or particular types of fear), nor do they offer explanations as to why the anxiolytic effect of alcohol appears more potent with some anxiety disorders than others.

There are at least several possible explanations for the differentially high relationship between excess alcohol use and social phobias. One simple possibility may be that situations that provoke social anxiety occur more often in settings where it is socially appropriate to drink. Thus the patient may simply "develop a habit" through repeated reinforcing experiences. A cycle of anxiety reduction by using alcohol may then become associated with the social situation, resulting in increased comfort (although sometimes accompanied by a perception of diminished social competence without the alcohol). In contrast, a simple phobia might be more easily managed by avoiding the feared object.

It may be that the anxiolytic effect of alcohol is more potent for certain anxiety disorders than others. We know that alcohol appears to affect the GABA-benzodiazepine chloride complex, apparently having an agonist-like action. However, our understanding of the neuronal mechanisms by which the different anxiety disorders are mediated is insufficient to explain a differential effect of alcohol on underlying structures or systems. Schneier et al. (1989) found higher rates of alcoholism in relatives of both alcoholic and nonalcoholic social phobia patients, and they suggested some sort of shared genetic susceptibility in the family. Munjack and Moss (1981) found that both social phobia and agoraphobia patients had higher risk of alcohol problems among family members than did those with simple phobia. The Schneier study offered the hypothesis that self-medication of "subsyndromal social anxiety" may occur.

Another possible explanation is that the anxiety-reducing effects of alcohol are stronger for anxiety states with substantial cognitive components (Kushner et al., 1990; Wilson, 1987). Both agoraphobia and social phobia are commonly conceptualized as having more cognitive components than other anxiety disorders, which may account for some of the higher rates of alcohol usage. Hull (1981) has argued that alcohol interferes with the specific cognitive process having to do with self-awareness, thus possibly lessening negative self-judgments. These negative self-statements appear to play a major role in perpetuating social anxiety.

Diagnosis and treatment in alcohol treatment settings

The accurate diagnosis of social phobia among patients being evaluated and treated for alcohol dependency and abuse is hindered by some of the same problems that occur in other settings. Patients who have lived with and accommodated to their symptoms over long periods of time may not perceive themselves as having a disorder. Thus the diagnosis will be missed unless they are asked about specific symptoms. Commonly, the degree of distress and dysfunction associated with social phobia is underestimated even when the disorder is recognized. Some professionals may believe that generalized social phobia is a personality trait or disorder, perhaps somewhere between shyness and avoidant personality. This view is frequently accompanied by the belief that there are no specific treatments, particularly not medication.

Additional factors may mitigate against recognition of social phobia in the alcohol treatment setting. Staff members may not be familiar with the specific diagnosis (many persons working in drug and alcohol treatment units do not have a traditional mental health background), or they may be unfamiliar with *DSM-III-R* diagnoses. Because anxiety is so commonly associated with alcohol withdrawal, it may be assumed that these symptoms are "normal" for the setting and do not need further exploration. When signs of social or occupational dysfunction are present, they are more likely to be attributed to the alcoholism than to the behavioral effects of social anxiety.

The common and often easily elicited pattern of drinking in anticipation of and during specific social events may be ignored because of a lack of belief in its relevance. Some programs adopt the philosophy that alcohol abuse and/or dependence is the sole or primary disorder and that a "self-medication" explanation, particularly if offered by the patient, is, at worst, an irrelevant "excuse," or at best, a misunderstanding on the patient's part. In the best drug and alcohol treatment programs, the notion of comorbidity (i.e., the possibility of a dual diagnosis) is seriously considered, but this practice is far from universal. In fact, we are unaware of any of our social phobia patients having been properly diagnosed in prior substance abuse treatment programs.

The treatment of alcohol-related problems, when comorbid with social phobia, can be hampered by social anxiety. For example, some patients are unable to participate in group therapy (often a part of treatment programs) due to their fear of speaking in small-group settings. In some instances, their reticence was viewed as resistance to treatment, and they were threatened with dismissal from the overall program. One of our patients was unable to regain his driver's license because he found the required group therapy intolerable, despite his repeated efforts to participate. Alcoholics Anonymous is based on a group format, and although most groups take great care not to pressure individuals to speak in front of the group, there is often subtle but strong peer pressure to do so. Patients with severe social phobia may find even entering a meeting room to be difficult. Thus traditional AA therapy may be unavailable to such patients.

Another common concern in alcohol treatment programs is the use of psychotropic medications. Some programs simply forbid all medications that are considered "mind altering." The apparent rationale is that psychiatric symptoms are due to the alcoholism and that psychotropic medications will interfere with treatment or serve as a "crutch." Some programs specifically disallow treatment with benzodiazepines. This prohibition appears to arise from the belief that benzodiazepines are strongly addicting (which is not true), and that persons with "addictive personalities" tend to more easily abuse them. It should be noted that the concept of addictive personality remains controversial. Furthermore, the benzodiazepines have low potential for abuse except when there is evidence of a history of drug abuse.

Another clinical observation commonly cited by some drug and alcohol specialists (which has not been objectively substantiated) is that benzodiazepines lead to an increased likelihood of alcohol relapse. Intuitively, it would make sense that if patients are self-medicating social anxiety with alcohol, then relief of these symptoms would enable them to participate more actively in treatment and thus avoid further drinking. Unfortunately, definitive studies of this issue are not available. Our experience suggests that there is much individual variation in this area and that medication decisions should be made on a case-by-case basis.

Given the high rate of anxiety disorders, as well as other psychiatric disorders found in patients in alcohol treatment settings, it is extremely important that adequate psychiatric evaluation be available for all patients. Accurate evaluation is sometimes difficult during the detoxification period because anxiety symptoms related to alcohol withdrawal may persist for the first 10-14 days. In such cases, subsequent evaluation may be needed. Decisions about concurrent versus sequential treatment of comorbid disorders can be made only after the specific disorders are recognized. Early in treatment, appropriate medications can be selected or, at the very least, specific cognitive-behavioral therapies can be started.

Management of alcohol-related problems in mental health settings

The excessive use of alcohol so commonly found with social phobia is also often overlooked in settings that treat social phobia. Patients who have used alcohol over long periods of time to self-medicate prior to social events may be so accustomed to this behavior that they do not see it as a problem; it has become ego-syntonic. For patients who admit to alcohol usage, a careful history regarding amount, setting, and pattern of intake is essential.

Socially anxious patients commonly drink before social events, such as dates, going to bars, company dinners, and parties. Conversely, unless the drinking problem is severe and chronic, many either do not drink when alone or do so infrequently. When asked directly about the effect of alcohol on their feelings of anxiety, most of our social phobia patients describe social anxiety reduction much more clearly and definitively than do patients with other types of anxiety, especially panic disorder or generalized anxiety.

The failure to recognize continued excessive alcohol use for social encounters can hamper therapeutic efforts. Abusive use tends to confuse the entire clinical picture. Patients who use alcohol heavily may report fluctuations in their anxiety symptoms both in intensity and in relationship to social stimuli. This reaction does not coincide with usual social phobia patterns, but is a common result of binge drinking and subsequent withdrawal effects. Cognitive and behavior therapies, which are mainstays in the treatment of social phobia, can be disrupted in various ways. Alcohol tends to alter cognitive states, and, as previously noted, may be one reason for self-medication. This cognitive alteration may interfere with therapeutic attempts to identify misconceptions or dysfunctional cognitions that need to be focused on and changed. The effectiveness of exposure experiences will also be complicated if the patient is drinking covertly. If the anxiety is dampened by alcohol, therapeutic habituation or desensitization to the situation appears less likely to occur. Patients may secretly attribute their successful endurance of the feared situation to the effects of the alcohol rather than to their own therapeutic success. Although patients are less likely to drink in the clinical setting, behavioral homework assignments—if done at all—may be especially undermined.

Finally, excessive alcohol use may be incompatible or even dangerous with medications used in the treatment of social phobia. Difficulties may arise secondary to additive effects such as increased sedation, excessive disinhibition, and diminished judgment. These effects may occur in combination with any psychotropic medication, but more commonly with monoamine oxidase inhibitors (MAOIs) or benzodiazepines. Patients who are drinking are also likely to forget doses of medication, resulting in further unevenness or irregularity in their clinical response. Occasionally, this problem is discovered when spouses or other relatives complain of the patient's response to medication. Interactions between drugs may also occur, particularly if the patient is being treated with MAOIs. Dangerous hypertensive episodes may occur in this circumstance.

Ideally, if an actual or potential alcohol problem exists for the social phobia patient, he or she would discontinue the use of alcohol. This can often be accomplished by carefully explaining the effects of alcohol and how it will interfere with satisfactory treatment. In fact, some patients are distinctly relieved to not need to self-medicate with alcohol because of unpleasant associated effects and consequences. If compliance is uncertain, and it is determined that the use of medication is desirable, one can prescribe a class of drugs least likely to cause difficulty. Of the three groups of medications with proven usefulness in the treatment of social phobia, the selective serotonin reuptake inhibitors (SSRIs—fluoxetine is the only one studied to date) would probably be the first choice, although evidence of their efficacy is somewhat less substantial than for MAOIs (phenelzine, tranylcypromine, moclobemide) or benzodiazepines (clonazepam) (Marshall, 1992).

If the social phobia is severe and other drugs have failed or cannot be used because of severe side effects, the benzodiazepines can be considered even though their use with alcoholic patients is controversial. In our clinic, if social phobia patients with a history of alcohol abuse or dependence are currently in alcohol treatment programs (and if their treaters concur) or if they have had a substantial period of abstinence (6-12 months), we occasionally use a benzodiazepine (usually clonazepam). However, the patient must engage in an ongoing social phobia treatment program and be monitored closely. Whenever possible, relatives are enlisted to support and monitor alcohol abstinence. Under these circumstances, some patients have had excellent success in the treatment of both of their disorders.

Not all social phobia patients who self-medicate with alcohol require a formal alcohol treatment program. Awareness of the problem, a good therapeutic relationship, and the occasional help of significant others can lead to successful treatment. Studies are increasingly finding that effective pretreatment of psychiatric problems is a good predictor of therapeutic response to drug and alcohol programs (McLellan, Luborsky, O'Brien, Barr, & Evans, 1986). If a separate alcohol treatment program is needed, substantial communication and teamwork increase the likelihood of a successful outcome.

References

Bibb, J.L., & Chambless, D.L. (1986). Alcohol use and abuse among diagnosed agoraphobics. *Behaviour Research and Therapy, 24,* 49-58.

Cappell, H., & Herman, C.P. (1972). Alcohol and tension reduction: A review. *Journal of Studies on Alcohol, 33,* 33-64.

Chambless, D.L., Cherney, J., Caputo, G.C., & Rheinstein, B.J.G. (1987). Anxiety disorders in alcoholism: A study with inpatient alcoholics. *Journal of Anxiety Disorders, 1,* 29-40.

Conger, J.J. (1956). Alcoholism: Theory, problem and challenge: II. Reinforcement theory and the dynamics of alcoholism. *Quarterly Journal of Studies on Alcohol, 17,* 296-305.

Hull J.G. (1981). A self-awareness model of the causes and effects of alcohol consumption. *Journal of Abnormal Psychology, 90,* 586-600.

Kessler, R.C., McGonagle, K.A., Zhao, S., Nelson, C.B., Hughes, M., Eshleman, S., Wittchen, H., & Kendler, K.S. (1994). Lifetime and 12-month prevalence of DSM-III-R psychiatric disorders in the United States. *Archives of General Psychiatry 51,* 8-19.

Kushner, M.G., Sher, K.J., & Beitman B.D. (1990). The relation between alcohol problems and the anxiety disorders. *American Journal of Psychiatry, 147,* 685-695.

Marshall, J.R. (1992). The psychopharmacology of social phobia. *Bulletin of the Menninger Clinic, 56*(2, Suppl. A), A42-A49.

McLellan, A.T., Luborsky, L., O'Brien, C.P., Barr, H.L., & Evans, F. (1986). Alcohol and drug abuse treatment in three different populations: Is there improvement and is it predictable? *American Journal of Drug and Alcohol Abuse, 12,* 101-102.

Mullaney, J.A., & Trippett, C.J. (1979). Alcohol dependence and phobias: Clinical description and relevance. *British Journal of Psychiatry, 135,* 565-573.

Munjack, D.J., & Moss, H.B. (1981). Affective disorders and alcoholism in families of agoraphobics. *Archives of General Psychiatry, 38,* 869-871.

Regier, D.A., Farmer, M.E., Rae, D.S., Locke, M.Z., Keith, S.J., Judd, L.L., & Goodwin F.K. (1990). Comorbidity of mental disorders with alcohol and other drug abuse: Results from the Epidemiologic Catchment Area (ECA) study. *Journal of the American Medical Association, 264,* 2511-2518.

Ross, H.E., Glaser, F.B., & Germanson, T. (1988). The prevalence of psychiatric disorders in patients with alcohol and other drug problems. *Archives of General Psychiatry 45,* 1023-1031.

Schneier, F.R., Martin, L.Y., Liebowitz, M.R., Gorman, J.M., & Fyer, A.J. (1989). Alcohol abuse in social phobia. *Journal of Anxiety Disorders, 3,* 15-23.

Sher, K.J. (1988). Stress response dampening. *Behaviour Research and Therapy, 26,* 369-381.

Smail, P., Stockwell, T., Canter, S., & Hodgson, R. (1984). Alcohol dependence and phobic anxiety states. *British Journal of Psychiatry, 144*, 53-57.

Thyer, B.A., Parrish, R.T., Himle, J., Cameron, O.G., Curtis, G.C., & Nesse, R.M. (1986). Alcohol abuse among clinically anxious patients. *Behaviour Research and Therapy, 24*, 357-359.

Wilson, G.T. (1987). Cognitive processes in addiction. *British Journal of Addiction, 82*, 343-353.

Winokur, G., & Holemon, E. (1963). Chronic anxiety neurosis: Clinical and sexual aspects. *Acta Psychiatrica Scandinavica, 39*, 384-412.

Woodruff, R.A., Jr., Guze, S.B., & Clayton, P.J. (1972). Anxiety neurosis among psychiatric outpatients. *Comprehensive Psychiatry, 13*, 165-170.

5. The Psychopharmacology of Social Phobia and Comorbid Disorders

Jerrold F. Rosenbaum, MD
Rachel A. Pollock, BA

Social phobia is characterized by a persistent fear of negative evaluation or scrutiny by others in social situations, resulting in excessive fear of humiliation or embarrassment (*DSM-III-R*, American Psychiatric Association, 1987). Exposure to the feared social situation or anticipation of the situation typically can produce an intense and immediate anxiety reaction, reinforcing the fear or avoidance of public activities. These social phobic situations may be limited to circumscribed events such as speaking in public or signing one's name in public, or may incorporate a pervasive fear encompassing a wide spectrum of generalized social situations.

Social phobia usually begins in adolescence and follows a chronic course with little spontaneous remission (Gorman & Papp, 1990; Liebowitz, Gorman, Fyer, & Klein, 1985). Epidemiological studies have indicated that approximately 2% of the adult U.S. population meet criteria for social phobia (Myers et al., 1984) and that a significant proportion of these individuals have at least one other comorbid psychiatric disorder.

Pharmacotherapy

Historically, pharmacotherapy has not been considered as first-line therapy for social phobia. Several factors have contributed to this view (Marshall, 1992). As the last anxiety disorder to be well studied, social phobia has pathophysiologic mechanisms that are not very well understood. Imprecise diagnostic assessment and a bias toward behavioral therapy for "phobias" have limited the use of drug therapy for social phobia. Discrete or performance social phobia has been considered a type of simple phobia that responds well to behavioral modification, while the generalized form has been confounded with avoidant personality disorder or viewed as a personality trait (i.e., as a manifestation of avoidant personality disorder or as a variant of severe shyness). In addition, some generalized social phobia patients, in clinical settings, are misdiagnosed as agoraphobia patients. However, recent attention to social phobia as a distinct clinical

Dr. Rosenbaum is director of the Outpatient Psychiatry Division and chief of the Clinical Psychopharmacology Unit at Massachusetts General Hospital in Boston, where Ms. Pollock is a senior research data analyst.

entity has redirected thought to an understanding of this syndrome as an independent Axis I disorder.

In recent years, clinical trials and case reports have documented the use of pharmacological therapy in social phobia. This evidence suggests that psychotropic agents can play a major role in the treatment of social phobia.

Beta-adrenergic blockers

There is a long tradition of using beta-adrenergic blocking agents for social phobia (Marshall, 1992). Theoretical support for this practice evolved from the James-Lange theory, which suggested that anxiety was a response to the perception of peripheral physiological sensations, as opposed to a phenomenon initiated in the central nervous system. By blocking such peripheral anxiety-provoking symptoms as sweating, palpitations, and tremors, beta-blockers were thought to reduce the central anxiety experience. The second factor supporting the use of beta-blockers in social phobia was the observed efficacy and common use of these agents among professional performing artists. Beta-blockers are thought to benefit performers by interfering with the generation and perception of peripheral symptoms (e.g., trembling) that may be interpreted as evidence of distress, which disturbs actual performance and consequently leads to anxiety.

Although beta-blocker efficacy has been documented in the professional artist who suffers from "performance anxiety" (Liebowitz et al., 1985), there have been few additional reports of beta-blocker therapy specifically for social phobia patients. In 1985 Liebowitz and colleagues reported an open clinical study of atenolol as a treatment for patients with social phobia. Five of the ten patients were reported to have experienced a "complete response," while four of the remaining five experienced a "moderate response." A double-blind, placebo-controlled trial, however, demonstrated that phenelzine was significantly superior to placebo, while atenolol resulted in an intermediate response that did not differ significantly from phenelzine or placebo (Liebowitz et al., 1992).

Monoamine oxidase inhibitors

In addition to their use in depression, monoamine oxidase inhibitors (MAOIs) have been observed to benefit patients with phobic anxiety. Liebowitz, Fyer, Gorman, Campeas, and Levin (1986) were prompted to investigate the efficacy of MAOIs in treating social phobia after phenelzine demonstrated anxiolytic properties in samples of patients with mixed agoraphobia-social phobia. In an open clinical trial, phenelzine was administered to 11 patients with social phobia; marked improvement was reported in seven patients, and moderate improvement was noted in the remaining four. These results were considered to reflect a property independent of phenelzine's antidepressant activity.

In a similar open clinical investigation with tranylcypromine, Versiani, Mundim, Nardi, and Liebowitz (1988) reported that of 29 patients treated with the drug for one year, 62% showed marked improvement and 17% showed moderate improvement. The authors reported findings that substantiate a true drug effect, including a high relapse rate following discontinuation of the MAOI, evidence of a dose-response curve, and latency to the appearance of therapeutic effects.

A double-blind controlled study comparing phenelzine, atenolol, and placebo in 85 social phobia patients was initiated by Liebowitz and colleagues (1988). After eight weeks, 64% of the phenelzine group was much improved or better, as compared with 30% of the atenolol patients and 23% of those in the placebo group. Further inspection of the data revealed that the superior effect of the MAOI over placebo or atenolol was limited to patients who had been classified as having the generalized form of social phobia, the subtype most likely to be high in interpersonal sensitivity. Where discrete performance anxiety was concerned, phenelzine and atenolol showed similar and moderate efficacy.

Of primary concern in managing a patient on MAOIs is compliance, particularly adherence to a low tyramine diet to prevent a hypertensive crisis. In light of this concern, moclobemide, a reversible inhibitor of the monoamine oxidase A enzyme that does not restrict dietary tyramine, holds promise for the treatment of social phobia. Versiani and colleagues (1992) conducted a double-blind, parallel group trial of moclobemide, phenelzine, and placebo in 78 subjects. The authors reported that 82% of the subjects receiving moclobemide and 92% of those receiving phenelzine were "almost asymptomatic" after 16 weeks. Of interest, moclobemide was reported to be better tolerated than phenelzine.

Benzodiazepines

The efficacy of benzodiazepines in treating other anxiety disorders suggested promise also in the management of social phobia. In 1988 Lydiard, Laraia, Howell, and Ballenger published case reports of four patients with the disorder who responded "moderately to markedly well" when treated with the triazolobenzodiazepine, alprazolam. Later that year Reich and Yates (1988) also reported efficacy of alprazolam in an open pilot study of 14 social phobia patients who also experienced improvement in six of nine examined avoidant personality traits (Reich, Noyes, & Yates, 1989). However, social phobia and avoidant behavior returned to baseline after alprazolam was discontinued.

Clonazepam has also been investigated as a treatment for social phobia. Reiter, Pollack, Rosenbaum, and Cohen (1990) reported that 9 of 11 social phobia patients experienced "clinically significant improvement" during treatment with clonazepam. The largest reported investigation of clonazepam (Davidson et al., 1993) is a double-blind study of 75 patients with social phobia. Over a 10-week course of treatment, 78% of those who received clonazepam reported amelioration of symptoms, while only 20% of the placebo group responded. This placebo response rate was "almost exactly" the same as the spontaneous recovery rate for social phobia reported in a community epidemiological study (Davidson et al., 1993).

Selective serotonin reuptake inhibitors

As a result of their efficacy, safety, and favorable side-effect profiles, the selective serotonin reuptake inhibitors (SSRIs) have been widely accepted as first-line treatment of depression and other disorders. This class of drugs is also being investigated as a potential treatment for social phobia. Three open clinical trials with fluoxetine have reported success. Schneier, Chin, Hollander, and Liebowitz (1992) found that 7 of 12 social phobia patients experienced a "moderate to marked" response to fluoxetine. Mean maximal dose was 25.7 mg for the responders and 25.0 mg for the nonresponders. Seven of the 12 subjects had comorbid disorders, and in general the response both of social phobia and of the comorbid disorder was favorable. In addition, several of the patients who responded to fluoxetine had failed previous medication trials.

In a second open clinical trial with fluoxetine, Black, Uhde, and Tancer (1992) reported that 10 of their 14 patients had "moderate or marked" improvement. Significant improvement was noted in 7 of 10 patients treated with fluoxetine alone, and in 3 of 4 who were treated with the SSRI added to another anxiolytic medication. Of note, all three patients who had previously been treated with phenelzine preferred fluoxetine to phenelzine.

In a third open clinical trial, Van Ameringen, Mancini, and Streiner (1993) noted that 10 of the 13 patients who completed the study exhibited a significant improvement from baseline. The responders were more likely to have been older at the onset of social phobia symptoms and had a shorter duration of illness. The major shortcomings of all three of these fluoxetine studies are the open design, lack of a control group, and potential confounding effects of comorbid conditions such as depression or other anxiety disorders.

Other medications

In addition to the clinical trials just described, several other pharmacological agents have been investigated for their potential roles in treating social phobia. An open trial of buspirone in 17 social phobia patients (Munjack et al., 1991) revealed that symptoms of generalized social phobia only partially responded to this anxiolytic, with few patients experiencing dramatic response. In a case report, clonidine was found useful with a social phobia patient with blushing attacks for whom other psychotropic agents had failed (Goldstein, 1987).

Comorbidity

Although several agents have probable efficacy in treating social phobia, the presence of comorbid conditions in psychopathology is a frequent obstacle to fully successful unimodal therapy. In the National Comorbidity Study (Kessler et al., 1994), 56% of the respondents with a history of at least one disorder had two or more disorders. Kessler and colleagues (1994) found a total lifetime prevalence of 13.3% for social phobia and a 12-month prevalence of 7.9% for social phobia. The clinician should consider patterns of comorbidity, the possible relationships between social phobia and other disorders, and their implications for clinical care.

Social phobia and other anxiety disorders
Rates of co-occurrence of social phobia with both Axis I and Axis II disorders are high; in particular, other anxiety disorders frequently co-occur with social phobia. Van Ameringen, Mancini, Styan, and Donison (1991) reported that 70% of a sample of social phobia patients suffered from at least one other anxiety disorder, including panic disorder (49.1%), generalized anxiety disorder (31.6%), simple phobia (19.3%), and obsessive-compulsive disorder (10.5%).

Furthermore, the majority of individuals suffering from *any* anxiety disorder experienced a degree of social anxiety, particularly a concern with being observed or humiliated (Rapee, Sanderson, & Barlow, 1988). The picture of anxiety disorders that emerges is consistent with an interplay of a physiological predisposition to anxiety and varying behavioral adaptations. This interaction often could generate the clinical picture of comorbid disorders.

Social phobia and panic disorder
Investigators have noted substantial comorbidity of panic disorder and social phobia (Amies, Gelder, & Shaw, 1983; Barlow, 1985; de Ruiter, Rijken, Garssen, van Schaik, & Kraaimaat, 1989; Mannuzza, Fyer, Liebowitz, & Klein, 1990; Reich, Noyes, & Yates, 1988; Reiter, Otto, Pollack, & Rosenbaum, 1991; Rosenbaum, Biederman, Hirsh-

feld, Bolduc, & Chaloff, 1991; Schneier, Johnson, Hornig, Liebowitz, & Weissman, 1992; Starcevic, Uhlenhuth, Kellner, & Pathak, 1992; Stein, Shea, & Uhde, 1989; Turner, Beidel, Borden, Stanley, & Jacob, 1991; Van Ameringen et al., 1991). One third to one half of panic disorder patients also suffer from social phobia symptoms (Barlow, 1985; de Ruiter et al., 1989; Mannuzza et al., 1990; Rosenbaum et al., 1988; Stein et al., 1989; Turner & Beidel, 1989). In one study (Stein et al., 1989), 46% of patients with *DSM-III-R* panic disorder had comorbid social phobia. Ninety-four percent of those patients also had suffered at least one major depressive episode; the social phobia preceded the depression in 69% of the cases. It has been noted that panic disorder patients with comorbid social phobia are "less assertive [and] have more dysfunctional attitudes" than patients without comorbid social phobia, which may predispose them to a history of depressive episodes (Reiter et al., 1991, p. 172). However, social phobia increases the risk for major depressive disorder independent of the presence of panic disorder (Stein & Uhde, 1988).

Reports of the temporal relationship of comorbid social phobia and panic disorder reveal that the social phobia typically has an earlier age of onset than panic disorder and agoraphobia (Barlow, 1985; de Ruiter et al., 1989). Van Ameringen et al. (1991) found that 17.9% of social phobia patients had onset of social phobia at the same time as that of panic disorder, while 60.7% had the onset of social phobia before panic disorder. This observation supports the hypothesis, elsewhere advanced, that some patients suffer an anxiety diathesis that manifests with a sequence of pathology from childhood anxiety disorder to adolescent onset social phobia and later onset of panic disorder (Rosenbaum, Biederman, Hirshfeld, Bolduc, & Chaloff, 1991; Rosenbaum, Biederman, Hirshfeld, Bolduc, Faraone, et al., 1991).

It has been suggested that the social avoidance of the person with comorbid social phobia and agoraphobia may be secondary to the desire to avoid the humiliation of a panic attack in the presence of others, as opposed to "true" social phobia (Liebowitz et al., 1985). The confusion of typology between social phobic and agoraphobic avoidance also extends to the misdiagnosis of some generalized social phobia patients as agoraphobia patients.

Munjack, Brown, and McDowell (1987) compared social phobia, panic disorder, and agoraphobia subjects on relative interpersonal sensitivity. Patients with social phobia scored highest on interpersonal sensitivity, while panic disorder patients were more sensitive to somatization factors. These conclusions support the distinction between social phobia and social anxiety that is secondary to the fear of embarrassment during a panic attack. In addition, agoraphobia patients tend to seek out the support of others to help assuage their anxiety, while social phobia patients are typically most comfortable when they are alone.

Social phobia and depression

The association between anxiety and depression was discussed as early as 1893 by Hecker and 1895 by Freud. Current research also indicates a high rate of comorbidity between the anxiety disorders, particularly panic disorder, and depression (Amies et al., 1983; Dilsaver, Qamar, & Del Medico, 1992; Kendler, Heath, Martin, & Eaves, 1986; Liebowitz et al., 1985, 1988; Reich et al., 1988; Reiter et al., 1991; Schneier, Johnson, et al., 1992; Stein, Tancer, Gelernter, Vittone, & Uhde, 1990; Van Ameringen et al., 1991; Weissman, 1990). This association with depression has been explained as reflecting: (1) the consequence of phobic avoidance and demoralization, (2) the co-occurrence of two separate disorders, or (3) a common biological diathesis (Brooks, Baltazar, & Munjack, 1989). Although depressive symptoms may emerge at any point in the course of social phobia, they may have onset concomitant with avoidance of normal social activities and impaired functioning in the work environment (Liebowitz, 1993; Liebowitz et al., 1985, 1992; Turner, McCanna, & Beidel, 1987). Stein et al. (1990) reported that 35% of patients with social phobia had experienced at least one episode of major depression. Comorbid dysthymic disorder has also been found in more than 15% of social phobia patients (Munjack et al., 1991; Van Ameringen et al., 1991). In more than 80% of cases of social phobia with comorbid depression, the depressive symptoms developed after the disabling social fear and avoidance became pronounced (Brooks et al., 1989; Turner et al., 1991).

Atypical depression versus rejection-sensitivity

There are features in common between atypical depression and social phobia suggesting that a single treatment might serve for the comorbid conditions (Liebowitz et al., 1986, 1988, 1992). One approach (Liebowitz et al., 1992) suggests that pathological social anxiety is a manifestation of an underlying biochemical dysregulation found both in atypical depressive patients and in generalized social phobia patients who express high interpersonal sensitivity to possible criticism or rejection from others. To avoid negative input from others, social phobia patients will minimize their interpersonal contacts as much as possible. In extreme situations, these individuals may avoid work, school, and any social contact outside extremely familiar conditions and individuals, resulting in extreme levels of disability. Similarly, the atypical depressive episode is triggered by situations involving rejection or criticism from important figures in an individual's life.

Studies have demonstrated MAOI efficacy in reducing interpersonal hypersensitivity, suggesting a specific biological substrate and leading to speculation that dopaminergic mechanisms play a role in MAOI efficacy in social phobia and atypical depression (Liebowitz et al., 1988, 1992). Support for this proposition is indicated by lower levels of the dopamine metabolite homovanillic acid in the cerebrospinal fluid of introverted as compared to more extraverted depressive patients (King et al., 1986), and by high rates of social phobia in patients with Parkinson's disease (Stein, Heuser, Juncos, & Uhde, 1990), a dopaminergic deficiency. Social phobia typically predates the parkinsonism. On the other hand, clinical reports suggest that SSRIs, similar to MAOIs, may also be effective in both atypical depression and social phobia.

Social phobia and additional Axis I disorders
Social phobia has also been associated with obsessive-compulsive disorder (OCD) (11%; Schneier, Johnson, et al., 1992), eating disorders (3.5%; Schwalberg, Barlow, Alger, & Howard, 1992), somatization disorder (1.9%; Schneier, Johnson, et al., 1992), and substance abuse (18-43%; Kushner, Sher, & Beitman, 1990; Otto, Pollack, Sachs, O'Neil, & Rosenbaum, 1992; Schneier, Johnson, et al., 1992; Turner et al., 1991; Van Ameringen et al., 1991). An investigation by Otto and colleagues (1992) revealed that 43% of panic disorder patients with comorbid social phobia also had a history of alcohol dependence, in comparison to 16% of patients without a diagnosis of social phobia. Almost 85% of those patients had onset of social phobia prior to the development of their alcohol problems. Attempts to self-medicate, to reduce anxiety cued in social situations where alcohol may be appropriate or highly available, or to alleviate the fear of negative social evaluation may underlie the high rates of alcohol abuse in this population (Mannuzza et al., 1990; Otto et al., 1992).

Behavioral inhibition:
Implications for an anxiety diathesis

The frequent co-occurrence of social phobia with such other disorders as depression and panic disorder suggests that, for some persons, there may be a common underlying predisposition or diathesis that manifests as the specific "disorders," as determined by other biological, environmental, or developmental factors. Recent studies of behavioral inhibition to the unfamiliar, the temperamental predisposition characterized by the tendency to excessive arousal and withdrawal from novelty, suggest that temperamental differences evident in early infancy may provide information about predisposition to developing anxiety pathology across the life cycle (Rosenbaum et al., 1992; Rosenbaum, Biederman, Hirshfeld, Bolduc, & Chaloff, 1991; Rosenbaum, Biederman, Hirshfeld, Bolduc, Faraone, et al., 1991). The ultimate manifestation of an anxiety disorder in childhood or adulthood may depend on the extent of the dysregulation inherited or the interaction of this predisposition with such environmental factors as parental psychopathology or adverse life events.

Rosenbaum and colleagues (1988) found that behavioral inhibition was highly prevalent in the offspring of adults with panic disorder and agoraphobia, but more than 30% of these adult panic disorder subjects also had a comorbid diagnosis of social phobia. In a further study (Rosenbaum, Biederman, Hirshfeld, Bolduc, Faraone, et al., 1991), our findings indicated that in comparison to normal controls, inhibited children had a significantly increased risk for multiple anxiety disorders, overanxious disorder, avoidant disorders, and phobic disorders. The phobic situations reported by the inhibited children were reminiscent of adult agoraphobia and social phobia. At a 3-year follow-up (Biederman et al., 1993), the inhibited children were also more likely than uninhibited children to meet criteria for avoidant disorder. According to Liebowitz and colleagues (1992), social phobia of childhood and adolescence may constitute a substantial proportion of what is now called overanxious disorder or avoidant disorder.

Social fears have also been found to be a major cause of school refusal and avoidant disorder in adolescents (Biederman, 1990). Our results indicate that the parents of behaviorally inhibited children often suffered from similar childhood psychopathologies themselves (Rosenbaum et al., 1992; Rosenbaum, Biederman, Hirshfeld, Bolduc, Faraone, et al., 1991). When psychopathology was assessed in the parents of the behaviorally inhibited children, there were significantly higher risks for adult social phobia as well as a childhood history of avoidant disorder and overanxious disorder. These results suggest that inhibited temperamental characteristics evident in childhood may be a precursor to the development of pathological anxiety later in life.

Impact of comorbidity on course of treatment

Patterns of comorbidity have important clinical and theoretical implications. The course and outcome for patients with concurrent additional diagnoses may be quite different from, and typically less satisfactory than, those of patients without comorbidity (Otto et al.,

1992; Sanderson, DiNardo, Rapee, & Barlow, 1990). Comorbidity may reflect more severe loading for psychopathology (Rosenbaum et al., 1992), which can in turn lead to increased disability and impairment of overall functioning. In a study by Turner et al. (1991), social phobia patients with an additional Axis I disorder had higher scores on several measures indicative of more severe anxiety.

In addition, depression ratings demonstrated that social phobia patients with any comorbid Axis I or Axis II disorder were significantly more depressed than those with social phobia alone. Reiter and colleagues (1991) investigated major depression in panic disorder patients with comorbid social phobia. As noted earlier, analyses revealed that panic disorder patients with comorbid social phobia had significantly higher measures of dysfunctional attitudes, social avoidance, and negative self-evaluation and lower scores on measures of assertiveness than those without social phobia. The panic disorder patients with comorbid social phobia were subsequently more likely to have a history of depression than patients without comorbid social phobia. The comorbid condition has also been associated with increased frequency of suicide attempts and higher rates of treatment-seeking than has uncomplicated social phobia (Johnson, Weissman, & Klerman, 1990; Schneier, Johnson, et al., 1992).

Treatment of the comorbid condition

Despite the prevalence and clinical significance of social phobia with comorbid conditions, the clinical trial literature offers poor guidance on treatment selection in the presence of comorbidity. Nonetheless, clinical experience that draws both on principles of patient management and on treatments with established efficacy for the comorbid conditions helps to guide the choice of pharmacological treatment of social phobia complicated by other disorders (see Table 1).

The clinical challenge

The clinical challenges in treating social phobia that is comorbid with other disorders include: (1) the need for systematic clinical assessment to identify and characterize comorbid disorders; (2) expectation of a more difficult treatment course, treatment resistance, and the likelihood of a less favorable outcome; (3) recognition that therapeutic efforts must address each individual disorder; thus the intensity of treatment may often be greater than for noncomorbid conditions; and (4) the necessity of extended continuation and maintenance treatment because relapse of one or more of the disorders is greater for comorbid conditions.

Principles of pharmacotherapy

Principles of pharmacotherapy for social phobia co-occurring with other psychiatric disorders include: (1) It is preferable, but rarely critical, to treat with a single agent when: (a) that agent is known to be efficacious for each disorder separately, and (b) comorbid disorders are felt to be clearly secondary to one disorder (e.g., social phobia complicating panic disorder or major depression); (2) co-pharmacy, when using compatible agents effective for individual disorders, is acceptable and frequently necessary; and (3) cognitive-behavioral therapy, especially group therapy, which is always appropriate as a treatment for social phobia and as an adjunct for partial or nonresponders to pharmacotherapy, should also be considered for comorbid social phobia.

Pharmacological strategies for social phobia and comorbid disorders

Panic disorder

Available evidence indicates that both panic disorder and social pho-

Table 1. *Pharmacological strategies for social phobia and comorbid disorders*

Social phobia and panic disorder/agoraphobia
1. High-potency benzodiazepine (clonazepam, alprazolam)
2. Monoamine oxidase inhibitor
3. Selective serotonin reuptake inhibitor
4. (?) Serotonergic tricyclic antidepressant (clomipramine)

Social phobia and depression
1. Monoamine oxidase inhibitor
2. Selective serotonin reuptake inhibitor
3. Selective serotonin reuptake inhibitor and benzodiazepine

Social phobia and obsessive-compulsive disorder
1. Selective serotonin reuptake inhibitor
2. Monoamine oxidase inhibitor
3. Clomipramine

Social phobia and alcoholism
1. Selective serotonin reuptake inhibitor
2. Reversible MAO-A inhibitor (moclobemide)
3. Buspirone and cognitive-behavioral therapy
4. Clonazepam

Social phobia and personality disorders
1. Monoamine oxidase inhibitor
2. Selective serotonin reuptake inhibitor
3. (?) Benzodiazepine

bia respond to MAOIs, SSRIs, and the high-potency benzodiazepines (HPBs), specifically clonazepam and probably alprazolam also. For incomplete responders to one agent for either condition or for the comorbid condition, HPBs can be combined with either class of anti-depressants. Tricyclic antidepressants (TCAs) appear less effective for social phobia (Liebowitz et al., 1992), but they will help alleviate the panic disorder condition and diminish social phobia symptoms that arise specifically as a complication of panic attacks. Although not yet studied with social phobia, the serotonergic TCA, clomipramine, may prove useful in the comorbid state as well.

Depression
Given the phenomenological similarities between atypical depression and social phobia, particularly in the feature of rejection-sensitivity, MAOIs are likely to be the most efficacious drug treatment for the comorbid state, but they are not the agents of first choice because of their relative side-effect burden and risks. The clinical first choice would be an SSRI, augmented if necessary by an HPB. As with panic disorder, the non-atypical major depression could be treated with a TCA, but the social phobia would likely require an additional agent or cognitive-behavioral therapy.

Obsessive-compulsive disorder
The prognosis of obsessive-compulsive disorder has changed dramatically since the introduction of SSRIs, which have demonstrated 50-60% efficacy in treating the condition during controlled trials (Carrasco, Hollander, Schneier, & Liebowitz, 1992). The SSRIs would therefore likely be the agents of first choice in treating social phobia with comorbid OCD, with MAOIs and clomipramine as suitable alternative treatments. Recent reports (Bodkin & White, 1989; Hewlett, Vinagradov, & Agras, 1992; Ross & Piggott, 1993) suggest clonazepam as an effective treatment for OCD; this agent could serve as either a single therapy or as part of a combined therapy.

Alcoholism
Pharmacotherapy of social phobia patients with existing substance abuse problems is more difficult because of the increased risk of abuse of prescribed medication and of the ingestion of alcohol during treatment. In agoraphobia and social phobia, alcohol problems appear likely to follow from attempts at self-medication of anxiety (Kushner et al., 1990). Alcohol use may be especially reinforcing for patients with social anxiety and social phobia who fear negative social evaluation, because alcohol intoxication appears to decrease sensitivity to

social feedback and to serve as a buffer against the negative evaluative components of anxiety (Otto et al., 1992).

Among the antidepressants, SSRIs rather than MAOIs (because of the risk of adverse interactions with some alcoholic beverages) would be first recommended. The problems associated with the use of traditional MAOIs in the social phobia patient with concomitant alcoholism may be minimized with the reversible inhibitors of MAO-A such as moclobemide (Liebowitz et al., 1992), SSRIs, and nonbenzodiazepine anxiolytics such as buspirone—coupled with cognitive-behavioral management. Nonetheless, when alcohol use is clearly in the service of self-medication, and when other strategies have not been successful, some patients may experience dramatic improvement with carefully monitored trials of clonazepam.

Personality disorders

The literature surrounding the treatment of social phobia and comorbid Axis II diagnoses is limited. A case study reported successful treatment of social phobia and avoidant personality disorder with a monoamine oxidase inhibitor (Deltito & Perugi, 1986). Later, Reich et al. (1989) conducted a study to examine the efficacy of alprazolam on avoidant personality traits in social phobia patients. For 9 of 14 patients, six of the measured avoidant traits improved with treatment; however, all traits, with the exception of avoiding social or occupational activities requiring interpersonal contact, returned to baseline levels after treatment was discontinued. Given the phenomenological overlap between social phobia and avoidant personality disorder, whether a separate "personality" disorder is being treated apart from symptoms of social phobia itself is doubtful.

Conclusion

Although social phobia is a distinct disorder, it is frequently comorbid with other psychiatric disorders. Concurrent pathology complicates the treatment and management of social phobia. A flexible approach to the pharmacology of social phobia and comorbid disorders that considers certain therapeutic principles will yield the best results. The addition of a cognitive-behavioral treatment also improves outcome and addresses negative self-evaluations, low assertiveness, and dysfunctional cognitive assumptions that may mediate both social phobia and comorbid conditions. Controlled trials of pharmacological treatment of social phobia and other specific comorbid psychopathological conditions are necessary.

References

American Psychiatric Association. (1987). *Diagnostic and statistical manual of mental disorders* (3rd ed., rev.). Washington, DC: Author.

Amies, P., Gelder, M., & Shaw, P. (1983). Social phobia: A comparative clinical study. *British Journal of Psychiatry, 142,* 174-179.

Barlow, D.H. (1985). The dimensions of anxiety disorders. In A.H. Tuma & J.D. Maser (Eds.), *Anxiety and the anxiety disorders* (pp. 479-500). Hillsdale, NJ: Erlbaum.

Biederman, J. (1990). The diagnosis and treatment of adolescent anxiety disorders. *Journal of Clinical Psychiatry, 51*(5, Suppl.), 20-26.

Biederman, J., Rosenbaum, J.F., Bolduc-Murphy, E.A., Faraone, S.V., Chaloff, J., Hirshfeld, D.R., & Kagan, J. (1993). A 3-year follow-up of children with and without behavioral inhibition. *Journal of the American Academy of Child and Adolescent Psychiatry, 32,* 814-821.

Black, B., Uhde, T.W., & Tancer, M.E. (1992). Fluoxetine for the treatment of social phobia [Letter to the editor]. *Journal of Clinical Psychopharmacology, 12,* 293-295.

Bodkin, J.A., & White, K. (1989). Clonazepam in the treatment of obsessive compulsive disorder associated with panic disorder in one patient. *Journal of Clinical Psychiatry, 50,* 265-266.

Brooks, R.B., Baltazar, P.L., & Munjack, D.J. (1989). Co-occurrence of personality disorders with panic disorder, social phobia, and generalized anxiety disorder: A review of the literature. *Journal of Anxiety Disorders, 3,* 259-285.

Carrasco, J.L., Hollander, E., Schneier, F.R., & Liebowitz, M.R. (1992). Treatment outcome of obsessive compulsive disorder with comorbid social phobia. *Journal of Clinical Psychiatry, 53,* 387-391.

Davidson, J.R.T., Potts, N., Richichi, E., Krishnan, R., Ford, S.M., Smith, R., & Wilson, W.H. (1993). Treatment of social phobia with clonazepam and placebo. *Journal of Clinical Psychopharmacology, 13,* 423-428.

de Ruiter, C., Rijken, H., Garssen, B., van Schaik, A., & Kraaimaat, F. (1989). Comorbidity among the anxiety disorders. *Journal of Anxiety Disorders, 3,* 57-68.

Deltito, J.A., & Perugi, G. (1986). A case of social phobia with avoidant personality disorder treated with MAOI. *Comprehensive Psychiatry, 27,* 255-258.

Dilsaver, S., Qamar, A.B., & Del Medico, V.J. (1992). Secondary social phobia in patients with major depression. *Psychiatry Research, 44,* 33-40.

Freud, S. (1962). On the grounds for detaching a particular syndrome from neurasthenia under the description "anxiety neurosis." In J. Strachey (Ed. and Trans.), *The standard edition of the complete psychological works of Sigmund Freud* (Vol. 3, pp. 85-117). London: Hogarth Press. (Original work published 1895)

Goldstein, S. (1987). Treatment of social phobia with clonidine. *Biological Psychiatry, 22,* 369-372.

Gorman, J.M., & Papp, L.A. (1990). Chronic anxiety: Deciding the length of treatment. *Journal of Clinical Psychiatry, 51*(1, Suppl.), 11-15.

Hecker, E. (1893). Über Iarvirte und abortive angstzustande bei neurasthenie zentralbl. *Nervenheilk, 133,* 565-572.

Hewlett, W.A., Vinogradov, S., & Agras, W.S. (1992). Clomipramine, clonazepam, and clonidine treatment of obsessive-compulsive disorder. *Journal of Clinical Psychopharmacology, 12,* 420-430.

Johnson, J., Weissman, M.M., & Klerman, G.L. (1990). Panic disorder, comorbidity, and suicide attempts. *Archives of General Psychiatry, 47,* 805-808.

Kendler, K.S., Heath, A., Martin, N.G., & Eaves, L.J. (1986). Symptoms of anxiety and depression in a volunteer twin population: The etiologic role of genetic and environmental factors. *Archives of General Psychiatry, 43,* 213-221.

Kessler, R.C., McGonagle, K.A., Zhao, S., Nelson, C.B., Hughes, M., Eshleman, S., Wittchen, H., & Kendler, K.S. (1994). Lifetime and 12-month prevalence of DSM-III-R psychiatric disorders in the United States. *Archives of General Psychiatry, 51,* 8-19.

King, R.J., Mefford, I.N., Wang, C., Murchison, A., Caligari, E.J., & Berger, P.A. (1986). CSF dopamine levels correlate with extraversion in depressed patients. *Psychiatry Research, 19,* 305-310.

Kushner, M.G., Sher, K.J., & Beitman, B.D. (1990). The relation between alcohol problems and the anxiety disorders. *American Journal of Psychiatry, 147,* 685-695.

Liebowitz, M.R. (1993). Depression with anxiety and atypical depression. *Journal of Clinical Psychiatry, 54*(2, Suppl.), 10-14.

Liebowitz, M.R., Fyer, A.J., Gorman, J.M., Campeas, R., & Levin, A. (1986). Phenelzine in social phobia. *Journal of Clinical Psychopharmacology, 6,* 93-98.

Liebowitz, M.R., Gorman, J.M., Fyer, A.J., Campeas, R., Levin, A., Sandberg, D., Hollander, E., Papp, L., & Goetz, D. (1988). Pharmacotherapy of social phobia: An interim report of a placebo-controlled comparison of phenelzine and atenolol. *Journal of Clinical Psychiatry, 49,* 252-257.

Liebowitz, M.R., Gorman, J.M., Fyer, A.J., & Klein, D.F. (1985). Social phobia: Review of a neglected anxiety disorder. *Archives of General Psychiatry, 42,* 729-736.

Liebowitz, M.R., Schneier, F., Campeas, R., Hollander, E., Hatterer, J., Fyer, A., Gorman, J., Papp, L., Davies, S., Gully, R., & Klein, D.F. (1992). Phenelzine vs atenolol in social phobia: A placebo-controlled comparison. *Archives of General Psychiatry, 49,* 290-300.

Lydiard, R.B., Laraia, M.T., Howell, E.F., & Ballenger, J.C. (1988). Alprazolam in the treatment of social phobia. *Journal of Clinical Psychiatry, 49,* 17-19.

Mannuzza, S., Fyer, A.J., Liebowitz, M.R., & Klein, D.F. (1990). Delineating the boundaries of social phobia: Its relationship to panic disorder and agoraphobia. *Journal of Anxiety Disorders, 4,* 41-59.

Marshall, J.R. (1992). The psychopharmacology of social phobia. *Bulletin of the Menninger Clinic, 56*(2, Suppl. A), A42-A49.

Munjack, D.J., Brown, R.A., & McDowell, D.E. (1987). Comparison of social anxiety in patients with social phobia and panic disorder. *Journal of Nervous and Mental Disease, 175,* 49-51.

Munjack, D.J., Bruns, J., Baltazar, P.L., Brown, R., Leonard, M., Nagy, R., Koek, R., Crocker, B., & Schafer, S. (1991). A pilot study of buspirone in the treatment of social phobia. *Journal of Anxiety Disorders, 5,* 87-98.

Myers, J.K., Weissman, M.M., Tischler, G.L., Holzer, C.E. III, Leaf, P.J., Orvaschel, H., Anthony, J.C., Boyd, J.H., Burke, J.D., Jr., Kramer, M., & Stoltzman, R. (1984). Six-month prevalence of psychiatric disorders in three communities: 1980 to 1982. *Archives of General Psychiatry, 41,* 959-967.

Otto, M.W., Pollack, M.H., Sachs, G.S., O'Neil, C.A., & Rosenbaum, J.F. (1992). Alcohol dependence in panic disorder patients. *Journal of Psychiatry Research, 26,* 29-38.

Rapee, R.M., Sanderson, W.C., & Barlow, D.H. (1988). Social phobia features across the DSM-III-R anxiety disorders. *Journal of Psychopathology and Behavioral Assessment, 10,* 287-299.

Reich, J., Noyes, R., & Yates, W. (1988). Anxiety symptoms distinguishing social phobia from panic and generalized anxiety disorders. *Journal of Nervous and Mental Disease, 176,* 510-513.

Reich, J., Noyes, R., & Yates, W. (1989). Alprazolam treatment of avoidant personality traits in social phobic patients. *Journal of Clinical Psychiatry, 50,* 91-95.

Reich, J., & Yates, W. (1988). A pilot study of treatment of social phobia with alprazolam. *American Journal of Psychiatry, 145,* 590-594.

Reiter, S.R., Otto, M.W., Pollack, M.H., & Rosenbaum, J.F. (1991). Major depression in panic disorder patients with comorbid social phobia. *Journal of Affective Disorders, 22,* 171-177.

Reiter, S.R., Pollack, M.H., Rosenbaum, J.F., & Cohen, L.S. (1990). Clonazepam for the treatment of social phobia. *Journal of Clinical Psychiatry, 51,* 470-472.

Rosenbaum, J.F., Biederman, J., Bolduc, E.A., Hirshfeld, D.R., Faraone, S.V., & Kagan, J. (1992). Comorbidity of parental anxiety disorders as risk for childhood-onset anxiety in inhibited children. *American Journal of Psychiatry, 149,* 475-481.

Rosenbaum, J.F., Biederman, J., Gersten, M., Hirshfeld, D.R., Meminger, S.R., Herman, J.B., Kagan, J., Reznick, J.S., & Snidman, N. (1988). Behavioral inhibition in children of parents with panic disorder and agoraphobia: A controlled study. *Archives of General Psychiatry, 45,* 463-470.

Rosenbaum, J.F., Biederman, J., Hirshfeld, D.R., Bolduc, E.A., & Chaloff, J. (1991). Behavioral inhibition in children: A possible precursor to panic disorder or social phobia. *Journal of Clinical Psychiatry, 51*(11, Suppl.), 5-9.

Rosenbaum, J.F., Biederman, J., Hirshfeld, D.R., Bolduc, E.A., Faraone, S.V., Kagan, J., Snidman, N., & Reznick, J.S. (1991). Further evidence of an association between behavioral inhibition and anxiety disorders: Results from a family study of children from a non-clinical sample. *Journal of Psychiatric Research, 25*(1/2), 49-65.

Ross, D.C., & Piggott, L.R. (1993). Clonazepam for OCD. *Journal of the American Academy of Child and Adolescent Psychiatry, 32,* 470-471.

Sanderson, W.C., DiNardo, P.A., Rapee, R.M., & Barlow, D.H. (1990). Syndrome comorbidity in patients diagnosed with a DSM-III-R anxiety disorder. *Journal of Abnormal Psychology, 99,* 308-312.

Schneier, F.R., Chin, S.J., Hollander, E., & Liebowitz, M.R. (1992). Fluoxetine in social phobia [Letter to the editor]. *Journal of Clinical Psychopharmacology, 12,* 62-63.

Schneier, F.R., Johnson, J., Hornig, C.D., Liebowitz, M.R., & Weissman, M.M. (1992). Social phobia: Comorbidity and morbidity in an epidemiologic sample. *Archives of General Psychiatry, 49,* 282-288.

Schwalberg, M.D., Barlow, D.H., Alger, S.A., & Howard, L.J. (1992). Comparison of bulimics, obese binge eaters, social phobics, and individuals with panic disorder on comorbidity across DSM-III-R anxiety disorders. *Journal of Abnormal Psychology, 101,* 675-681.

Starcevic, V., Uhlenhuth, E.H., Kellner, R., & Pathak, D. (1992). Patterns of comorbidity in panic disorder and agoraphobia. *Psychiatry Research, 42,* 171-183.

Stein, M.B., Heuser, I.J., Juncos, J.L., & Uhde, T.W. (1990). Anxiety disorders in patients with Parkinson's disease. *American Journal of Psychiatry, 147,* 217-220.

Stein, M.B., Shea, C.A., & Uhde, T.W. (1989). Social phobic symptoms in patients with panic disorder: Practical and theoretical implications. *American Journal of Psychiatry, 146,* 235-238.

Stein, M.B., Tancer, M.E., Gelernter, C.S., Vittone, B.J., & Uhde, T.W. (1990). Major depression in patients with social phobia. *American Journal of Psychiatry, 147,* 637-639.

Stein, M.B., & Uhde, T. (1988). Panic disorder and major depression: A tale of two syndromes. *Psychiatric Clinics of North America, 11,* 441-461.

Turner, S.M., & Beidel, D.C. (1989). Social phobia: Clinical syndrome, diagnosis, and comorbidity. *Clinical Psychology Review, 9,* 3-18.

Turner, S.M., Beidel, D.C., Borden, J.W., Stanley, M.A., & Jacob, R.G. (1991). Social phobia: Axis I and II correlates. *Journal of Abnormal Psychology, 100,* 102-106.

Turner, S.M., McCanna, M., & Beidel, D.C. (1987). Validity of the Social Avoidance and Distress and Fear of Negative Evaluation scales. *Behaviour Research and Therapy, 25,* 113-115.

Van Ameringen, M., Mancini, C., & Streiner, D.L. (1993). Fluoxetine efficacy in social phobia. *Journal of Clinical Psychiatry, 54,* 27-32.

Van Ameringen, M., Mancini, C., Styan, G., & Donison, D. (1991). Relationship of social phobia with other psychiatric illness. *Journal of Affective Disorders, 21,* 93-99.

Versiani, M., Mundim, F.D., Nardi, A.E., & Liebowitz, M.R. (1988). Tranylcypromine in social phobia. *Journal of Clinical Psychopharmacology, 8,* 279-283.

Versiani, M., Nardi, A.E., Mundim, F.D., Alves, A.B., Liebowitz, M.R., & Amrein, R. (1992). Pharmacotherapy of social phobia: A controlled study with moclobemide and phenelzine. *British Journal of Psychiatry, 161,* 353-360.

Weissman, M.M. (1990). Evidence for comorbidity of anxiety and depression: Family and genetic studies of children. In J.D. Maser & C.R. Cloninger (Eds.), *Comorbidity of mood and anxiety disorders* (pp. 349-365). Washington, DC: American Psychiatric Press.

6. Psychotherapy and Integrated Treatment of Social Phobia and Comorbid Conditions

W. Walter Menninger, MD

Identified as a clinical entity nearly three decades ago (Marks, 1970; Marks & Gelder, 1966), social phobia was first included in the formal psychiatric nomenclature in 1980 with *DSM-III* (American Psychiatric Association, 1980). The clinical picture of this condition is a persistent and exaggerated fear of situations where one might be observed, scrutinized, or evaluated by others. This fear of humiliation or embarrassment prompts bodily sensations associated with anxiety and cognitive and behavioral symptoms in the sufferer. Common fears of socially phobic persons involve performing activities in public, such as speaking, eating, signing one's name, and using a lavatory; these fears also include being watched while doing something, being introduced, being stared at, or being the center of attention (Marshall, 1993; Uhde & Tancer, 1991). The worry and anxiety associated with these activities may lead to impairment for weeks or months in anticipation of a known future social event.

In the years since social phobia was formally recognized in the nomenclature, epidemiological studies have found a lifetime incidence in 2-3% of the United States population (Davidson, 1993). In a careful review of data from four U.S. communities among more than 13,000 adults from the Epidemiologic Catchment Area (ECA) study, almost 70% of the subjects with social phobia were female, younger, of lower socioeconomic status, less well educated, and less likely to be married. The mean reported age of onset was 15.5 years, with onset after age 25 uncommon (Schneier, Johnson, Hornig, Liebowitz, & Weissman, 1992).

If social phobia is not treated, its consequences can include academic underperformance, vocational limitations, social impairment, financial dependence, and excessive medical evaluations. In addition, one may see depression, agoraphobia, suicidal ideation, and the use of alcohol or other substances to self-medicate (Ross, 1993). Of the ECA subjects identified as having social phobia, only 31% were without some comorbid clinical disorder (Schneier et al., 1992). The most common comorbid conditions were simple phobia (59.0%) and agoraphobia (44.9%). The next most common conditions were alcohol

---

Dr. Menninger is president and chief executive officer, The Menninger Clinic, Topeka, Kansas.

abuse (18.8%), major depression (16.6%), drug abuse (13.0%), dysthymia (12.5%), and obsessive-compulsive disorder (11.1%). The rate of suicidal ideation was elevated in subjects with uncomplicated social phobia as well as in persons with comorbid social phobia. Schneier et al. (1992) concluded, "The high rate of comorbid disorders that usually occurred after the onset of social phobia suggests that social phobia may be a risk factor for additional psychiatric disorders" (pp. 285-286).

A Canadian study of 57 social phobia patients found that 70.2% suffered from at least one other anxiety disorder in their lifetime, and an equivalent percentage manifested a mood disorder, particularly major depression, at some point during their lifetime. The social phobia predated any episode of mood or other anxiety disorder, suggesting that social phobia may predispose individuals to other psychiatric illnesses (Van Ameringen, Mancini, Styan, & Donison, 1991).

Social phobia is often accompanied not only by Axis I but also by Axis II (personality) disorders. At the Western Psychiatric Institute in Pittsburgh, Turner, Beidel, Borden, Stanley, and Jacob (1991) carefully studied a sample of 71 patients with a diagnosis of social phobia. Forty-three percent of the patients were found to have one or more secondary Axis I diagnoses, while 37% had a secondary Axis II disorder. The most common comorbid Axis I diagnoses were generalized anxiety disorder (33.3%) and simple phobia (11.1%), followed by dysthymic disorder, panic disorder, major depressive disorder, obsessive-compulsive disorder, and substance abuse. Somewhat more than half of the patients with an Axis I diagnosis also had evidence of an Axis II disorder. The most prevalent Axis II diagnoses were avoidant personality disorder (22.1%) and obsessive-compulsive personality disorder (13.2%). Furthermore, 52.9% of the patients had a subthreshold diagnosis for avoidant personality disorder, and 48.5% had a subthreshold diagnosis for obsessive-compulsive personality disorder.

Treatment perspectives

In the previous chapters, several therapeutic perspectives have been presented regarding social phobia and comorbid conditions—psychodynamic, cognitive-behavioral, and psychopharmacological—with particular reference to the overlap between these conditions and other anxiety disorders and alcohol abuse. Clearly, the first step toward effective treatment is the recognition of this disorder and an appreciation for its impact on the sufferer. As Zerbe (1995) has observed, "Understanding and mastering a disorder is predicated on first recognizing that it is an affliction and then attempting to allay suffering it has caused with available therapeutics" (p. 1). Jerilyn Ross (1991), identified as a "consumer" and president of the Anxiety Disorders Association of America, decried the underdiagnosis and lack of understanding about this disorder:

It is ... apparent that there is a lack of public awareness and a lack of clinical knowledge among health care professionals about social phobia.... Many [sufferers tell] heartrending stories of their own plight ... describing the frustration of running from one doctor to the next without ever having been given a proper diagnosis or having received help, of missed career and family opportunities, of turning to alcohol, of having suffered bouts of depression, and of suicide ideation and attempts. (p. 440)

In the past decade, a variety of therapeutic interventions have been efficacious in the treatment of social phobia as well as for many of the conditions occurring in connection with social phobia. When the diagnosis of social phobia is made, the clinician may consider a range of psychotherapeutic and psychopharmacological approaches—all outlined in the preceding chapters. In a study sponsored by the National Institute of Mental Health, Gelernter et al. (1991) compared the outcomes of cognitive-behavioral techniques and pharmacotherapy for social phobia and concluded that both treatment approaches

are effective treatments, when combined with exposure, for some patients who are suffering with this disorder. Both pharmacotherapy and psychotherapy can be associated with marked cognitive and behavioral changes, but no single treatment can yet be designated as most effective. Thus, depending on the training and inclination of the clinician and preferences of the patient, it would be reasonable to use any of these modalities. The only unreasonable choice would be a decision not to treat. (p. 944)

With regard to specific therapeutic approaches, Uhde and Tancer (1991) reviewed reports of the efficacy of social skills training, relaxation training, exposure, and cognitive restructuring in patients with social phobia. However, they observed that different types of therapy under different formats (group or individual) and time frames (6-14 weeks) complicate the analysis of these studies: "While several of the studies reported superior results of one form of behavioral or cognitive therapy over another, differences in patient selection, outcome measure used, and duration and intensity of treatment make it premature to conclude that one form ... is superior to any other" (p. 246).

New insights regarding the effectiveness of psychotherapy for patients with social phobia should come from research in process at the University of California, San Francisco, Center for the Study of Neuroses, funded by the John D. and Catherine T. MacArthur Foundation. This project, under the direction of Horowitz and Stinson (1991), is focusing on how people process and adapt to recent traumatic events that precipitate symptom formation. The current main study explores two psychopathological syndromes: pathological grief and social phobia. The researchers noted that patients with either condition often change during a brief psychotherapy: "In the safety of a therapeutic relationship the person may reduce purposive unconscious controls or consciously override them" (p. 109). They also found that neither classical psychoanalytic theory nor cognitive theory satisfactorily explains the psychological process that takes place.

Principles of integrated treatment

Previously, I (1992) have outlined eight operating principles to be considered by the clinician for an integrated treatment of anxiety disorders (see Table 1). Those principles are equally applicable in addressing the treatment of comorbid conditions with social phobia. As noted in principle 2, it is essential to make a careful differential diagnosis, and to attend to significant comorbid conditions in the treatment plan.

Patients with social phobia often ask for medication to help them deal with particular situations. But, as suggested by Marshall (1991), before such medication is prescribed, patients should be told that some performance discomfort is "normal." They should also be encouraged to desensitize themselves to these experiences by controlled exposure. If the problem is one of public speaking, for example, the patient could be encouraged to participate in a toastmaster's club or to take a course designed to increase mastery and build confidence while improving speaking skills.

The use of medication should be based on how well the patient is able to tolerate discomfort and the consequences of the patient's inability to perform in a given social situation. Davidson, Ford, Smith, and Potts (1991) suggested that "in evaluating a particular treatment, it is important not to lose sight of three critical questions: (1) What is the cost of the untreated illness? (2) What is the impact of successful treatment on the quality of life? (3) What are the risks of treatment?" (pp. 19-20). These questions may help point to one or another therapeutic intervention that is appropriate for a given patient—recognizing that for these conditions, any of several treatment options may be

Table 1. *Principles of integrated treatment for anxiety disorders*

1. *Anxiety in the patient can provoke anxiety in the therapist.*
   The urgency felt by the patient resonates with the physician's training to take remedial action to relieve discomfort and anguish.

2. *A careful differential diagnosis can help identify and address the problem of comorbidity.*
   Recognition of a secondary diagnostic issue may come only as the patient fails to respond effectively to treatment for the anxiety.

3. *The anxiety disorder is often not initially recognized as such.*
   Patients frequently seek help for physical symptoms from an internist or family practitioner who searches for a physical explanation for the problem.

4. *The patient should be reassured that the symptoms are real.*
   The patient may not feel the symptoms are valid or real if another physician has said "they're all in your head." The patient needs to be validated as having a known and diagnosable illness.

5. *The patient should be helped to accept the condition as a psychiatric illness.*
   Patients who can accept their illness as psychiatric will be more receptive to taking psychotropic medication. Otherwise, they may resist taking medication.

6. *Symptomatic relief may be essential before psychological work can proceed.*
   Effective treatment involves a two-stage approach, with medication to relieve acute anxiety, after which brief or open-ended psychotherapy and behavioral therapy may be used to facilitate the patient's capacity to deal with the anxiety and address the underlying problems.

7. *Symptomatic relief is facilitated by enhancing the patient's confidence about being able to remain in control.*
   Techniques to enhance an individual's sense of being in control diminish anxiety. Cognitive-behavioral approaches typically incorporate various methods of anxiety control, including distraction, coping self-statements, paradoxical intention, relaxation, and meditation.

8. *A search should be made to determine the underlying cause; until it is recognized, symptoms may persist.*
   A persistent and careful search usually enables the treater to identify a precipitating incident or conflict. If that is effectively addressed, the need for additional treatment or medication may be markedly reduced. Often, the patient may have a strong psychological reason to deny the incident or conflict and to avoid seeing the link between exacerbation of the anxiety disorder and the stressors. The key may be a symbolic reexperiencing or association with an initial trauma, which often is related to a disrupted relationship or present or past abuse.

(Adapted from Menninger, 1992, pp. A66-A68)

equally efficacious. Of course, if the clinician has exceptional confidence in one or another proven therapy for the illness, that confidence will have a beneficial effect on the patient. The challenge to the clinician is to identify the treatment that best fits a given patient, consistent with the aforementioned operating principles.

References

American Psychiatric Association. (1980). *Diagnostic and statistical manual of mental disorders* (3rd ed.). Washington, DC: Author.

Davidson, J.R.T. (1993). Social phobia in review: 1993. *Journal of Clinical Psychiatry, 54*(12, Suppl.), 3-4.

Davidson, J.R.T., Ford, S.M., Smith, R.D., & Potts, N.L.S. (1991). Long-term treatment of social phobia with clonazepam. *Journal of Clinical Psychiatry, 52*(11, Suppl.), 16-20.

Gelernter, C.S., Uhde, T.W., Cimbolic, P., Arnkoff, D.B., Vittone, B.J., Tancer, M.E., & Bartko, J.J. (1991). Cognitive-behavioral and pharmacological treatments of social phobia: A controlled study. *Archives of General Psychiatry, 48,* 938-945.

Horowitz, M.J., & Stinson, C. (1991) University of California, San Francisco Center for the Study of Neuroses: Program on conscious and unconscious mental processes. In L.E. Beutler & M. Crago (Eds.), *Psychotherapy research* (pp. 107-114). Washington, DC: American Psychological Association.

Marks, I.M. (1970). The classification of phobic disorders. *British Journal of Psychiatry, 116,* 377-386.

Marks, I.M., & Gelder, M.C. (1966). Different ages of onset in varieties of phobia. *American Journal of Psychiatry, 123,* 218-221.

Marshall, J.R. (1991). Social phobia: Helping patients who are disabled by fear. *Postgraduate Medicine, 90,* 187-189, 192, 194.

Marshall, J.R. (1993). Social phobia: An overview of treatment strategies. *Journal of Clinical Psychiatry, 54,* 165-171.

Menninger, W.W. (1992). Integrated treatment of panic disorder and social phobia. *Bulletin of the Menninger Clinic, 56*(2, Suppl. A), A61-A70.

Ross, J. (1991). Social phobia: The Anxiety Disorders Association of America helps raise the veil of ignorance. *Journal of Clinical Psychiatry, 52*(11, Suppl.), 43-47.

Ross, J. (1993). Social phobia: The consumer's perspective. *Journal of Clinical Psychiatry, 54*(12, Suppl.), 5-9.

Schneier, F.R., Johnson, J., Hornig, C.D., Liebowitz, M.R., & Weissman, M.M. (1992). Social phobia: Comorbidity and morbidity in an epidemiologic sample. *Archives of General Psychiatry, 49,* 282-288.

Turner, S.M., Beidel, D.C., Borden, J.W., Stanley, M.A. & Jacob, R.G. (1991). Social phobia: Axis I and II correlates. *Journal of Abnormal Psychology, 100,* 102-106.

Uhde, T.W., & Tancer, M.E. (1991). Social phobia. In B.D. Beitman & G.L. Klerman (Eds.), *Integrating pharmacotherapy and psychotherapy* (pp. 231-252). Washington, DC: American Psychiatric Press.

Van Ameringen, M., Mancini, C., Styan, G., & Donison, D. (1991). Relationship of social phobia with other psychiatric illness. *Journal of Affective Disorders, 21,* 93-99.

Zerbe, K.J. (1995). Uncharted waters: Psychodynamic considerations in the diagnosis and treatment of social phobia. In W.W. Menninger (Ed.), *Fear of humiliation: Integrated treatment of social phobia and comorbid conditions* (pp. 1-17). Northvale, NJ: Aronson.

Index